Head, Eyes, Ears, Nose, and Throat Emergencies

Editors

ALISA M. GIBSON
KIP R. BENKO

EMERGENCY MEDICINE CLINICS OF NORTH AMERICA

www.emed.theclinics.com

Consulting Editor
AMAL MATTU

May 2013 • Volume 31 • Number 2

ELSEVIER

1600 John F. Kennedy Boulevard • Suite 1800 • Philadelphia, Pennsylvania, 19103-2899

http://www.theclinics.com

EMERGENCY MEDICINE CLINICS OF NORTH AMERICA Volume 31, Number 2
May 2013 ISSN 0733-8627, ISBN-13: 978-1-4557-7083-0

Editor: Patrick Manley
Developmental Editor: Donald Mumford

Emergency Medicine Clinics of North America (ISSN 0733-8627) is published quarterly by Elsevier Inc., 360 Park Avenue South, New York, NY, 10010-1710. Months of issue are February, May, August, and November. Business and Editorial Offices: 1600 John F. Kennedy Boulevard, Suite 1800, Philadelphia, PA 19103-2899. Customer Service Office: 6277 Sea Harbor Drive, Orlando, FL 32887-4800. Periodicals postage paid at New York, NY, and additional mailing offices. Subscription prices are $149.00 per year (US students), $298.00 per year (US individuals), $507.00 per year (US institutions), $211.00 per year (international students), $428.00 per year (international individuals), $609.00 per year (international institutions), $211.00 per year (Canadian students), $368.00 per year (Canadian individuals), and $609.00 per year (Canadian institutions). International air speed delivery is included in all *Clinics'* subscription prices. All prices are subject to change without notice. **POSTMASTER:** Send address changes to *Emergency Medicine Clinics of North America*, Elsevier Periodicals Customer Service, 11830 Westline Industrial Drive, St. Louis, MO 63146. Customer Service (orders, claims, online, change of address): Elsevier Periodicals Customer Service, 11830 Westline Industrial Drive, St. Louis, MO 63146. Tel: 1-800-654-2452 (U.S. and Canada); 314-453-7041 (outside U.S. and Canada). Fax: 314-453-5170. E-mail: journalscustomerservice-usa@elsevier.com (for print support); journalsonlinesupport-usa@elsevier.com (for online support).

Reprints. For copies of 100 or more of articles in this publication, please contact the Commercial Reprints Department, Elsevier Inc., 360 Park Avenue South, New York, NY 10010-1710. Tel.: 212-633-3812; Fax: 212-462-1935; E-mail: reprints@elsevier.com.

Emergency Medicine Clinics of North America is covered in *MEDLINE/PubMed (Index Medicus), Current Contents/Clinical Medicine, EMBASE/Excerpta Medica, BIOSIS, SciSearch, CINAHL, ISI/BIOMED,* and *Research Alert.*

Printed and bound by CPI Group (UK) Ltd, Croydon, CR0 4YY
Transferred to Digital Printing, 2013

Contributors

CONSULTING EDITOR

AMAL MATTU, MD
Professor and Vice Chair, Department of Emergency Medicine, University of Maryland School of Medicine, Baltimore, Maryland

EDITORS

ALISA M. GIBSON, MD, DMD
Clinical Assistant Professor, Department of Emergency Medicine, University of Maryland School of Medicine, Baltimore, Maryland

KIP R. BENKO, MD, FACEP
Clinical Assistant Professor, Department of Emergency Medicine, University of Pittsburgh School of Medicine, Pittsburgh, Pennsylvania

AUTHORS

MATTHEW A. ARMSTRONG, MD, MBA
Staff Emergency Physician, Captain USAF, Mike O'Callaghan Federal Hospital, Nellis Air Force Base, Las Vegas, Nevada

KIM A. BOSWELL, MD
Fellow, Surgical Critical Care, Shock Trauma Center, Baltimore, Maryland

ANGELA R. CIRILLI, MD, RDMS
Assistant Professor of Emergency Medicine, Hofstra North Shore-LIJ School of Medicine; Department of Emergency Medicine, North Shore University Hospital, Long Island Jewish Hospital, Manhasset, New York

KEITH CONOVER, MD, FACEP
Clinical Assistant Professor, Department of Emergency Medicine, University of Pittsburgh, Pittsburgh, Pennsylvania

KATHLEEN COWLING, DO, MS
Emergency Medicine Faculty, Synergy Medical Education Alliance, Saginaw, Michigan; Clinical Professor, College of Human Medicine, Michigan State University, Grand Rapids, Michigan

JONATHON P. DEIBEL, MD
Emergency Medicine Resident, Synergy Medical Education Alliance, Saginaw, Michigan; Clinical Instructor, College of Human Medicine, Michigan State University, Grand Rapids, Michigan

ALISA M. GIBSON, MD, DMD
Clinical Assistant Professor, Department of Emergency Medicine, University of Maryland
School of Medicine, Baltimore, Maryland

ALAN HODGDON, MD, MBA, FACEP
Clinical Assistant Professor, Department of Emergency Medicine, University of Pittsburgh
School of Medicine, Pittsburgh, Pennsylvania

ZACHARY A. KASPEREK, MD
Resident, Emergency Medicine Residency, University of Pittsburgh, Pittsburgh,
Pennsylvania

JOSHUA B. MOSKOVITZ, MD, MPH
Assistant Professor of Emergency Medicine, Department of Emergency Medicine,
North Shore University Hospital, Hofstra North Shore-Long Island Jewish
School of Medicine, Manhasset, New York

JOHN M. MURRAY, MD, FACEP
Attending Physician, Department of Emergency Medicine, Miles Memorial Hospital,
Lincoln County Health, Damariscotta, Maine

GARY F. POLLOCK, MD, FACEP
Emergency Medicine Residency, Associate Program Director, University of Pittsburgh;
Attending Physician, UPMC Mercy Hospital, Pittsburgh, Pennsylvania

VICTORIA M. ROMANIUK, MD
Visiting Instructor, Academic Emergency Medicine Fellow and Chief Resident,
Department of Emergency Medicine, University of Maryland School of Medicine,
Baltimore, Maryland

FRANK SABATINO, MD
Assistant Professor of Emergency Medicine, Department of Emergency Medicine,
North Shore University Hospital, Hofstra North Shore-Long Island Jewish
School of Medicine, Manhasset, New York

SARAH K. SOMMERKAMP, MD, RDMS
Assistant Professor, Department of Emergency Medicine, University of Maryland
School of Medicine, Baltimore, Maryland

MICHAEL A. TURTURRO, MD
Associate Professor of Emergency Medicine, University of Pittsburgh School of Medicine;
Chief of Emergency Services, Department of Emergency Medicine, UPMC Mercy
Hospital, Pittsburgh, Pennsylvania

Contents

EMERGENCY MEDICINE
CLINICS OF NORTH AMERICA

**DOWNLOAD
Free App!**

Review Articles
THE CLINICS

NOW AVAILABLE FOR YOUR iPhone and iPad

PROGRAM OBJECTIVE

The goal of *Emergency Medicine Clinics of North America* is to keep practicing emergency medicine physicians and emergency medicine residents up to date with current clinical practice in emergency medicine by providing timely articles reviewing the state of the art in patient care.

TARGET AUDIENCE

All practicing physicians and healthcare professionals who provide patient care utilizing findings from *Emergency Medicine Clinics of North America*.

LEARNING OBJECTIVES

Upon completion of this activity, participants will be able to:
1. Discuss emergency management of the sore throat and salivary glands.
2. Describe the evaluation and management of oral lesions in the emergency department.
3. Review nerve blocks of the face, management of facial fractures, and management of facial wounds.

ACCREDITATION

The Elsevier Office of Continuing Medical Education (EOCME) is accredited by the Accreditation Council for Continuing Medical Education (ACCME) to provide continuing medical education for physicians.

The EOCME designates this journal-based CME activity for a maximum of 12 *AMA PRA Category 1 Credit*(s)™. Physicians should claim only the credit commensurate with the extent of their participation in the activity.

All other health care professionals completing continuing education credit for this activity will be issued a certificate of participation.

DISCLOSURE OF CONFLICTS OF INTEREST

The EOCME assesses conflict of interest with its instructors, faculty, planners, and other individuals who are in a position to control the content of CME activities. All relevant conflicts of interest that are identified are thoroughly vetted by EOCME for fair balance, scientific objectivity, and patient care recommendations. EOCME is committed to providing its learners with CME activities that promote improvements or quality in healthcare and not a specific proprietary business or a commercial interest.

The planning committee, staff, authors and editors listed below have identified no financial relationships or relationships to products or devices they or their spouse/life partner have with commercial interest related to the content of this CME activity:

Matthew A. Armstrong, MD, MBA; Kim A. Boswell, MD; Angela R. Cirilli, MD, RDMS; Keith Conover, MD, FACEP; Kathleen Cowling, DO, MS; Jonathon P. Deibel, MD; Alisa M Gibson, MD, DMD; Alan Hodgdon, MD, MBA, FACEP; Zachary A. Kasperek, MD; Indu Kumari; Sandy Lavery; Patrick Manley; Amal Mattu, MD; Kristen McFarlane; Jill McNair; Joshua B. Moskovitz, MD, MPH; John M. Murray, MD, FACEP; Gary F. Pollock, MD; Victoria M. Romaniuk, MD; Frank Sabatino, MD; Sarah K. Sommerkamp, MD, RDMS; and Michael A. Turturro, MD.

The planning committee, staff, authors and editors listed below have identified financial relationships or relationships to products or devices they or their spouse/life partner have with commercial interest related to the content of this CME activity:

Kip R. Benko, MD's spouse has an employment affiliation with the Dental Box Company.

UNAPPROVED/OFF-LABEL USE DISCLOSURE

The EOCME requires CME faculty to disclose to the participants:
1. When products or procedures being discussed are off-label, unlabelled, experimental, and/or investigational (not US Food and Drug Administration (FDA) approved); and
2. Any limitations on the information presented, such as data that are preliminary or that represent ongoing research, interim analyses, and/or unsupported opinions. Faculty may discuss information about pharmaceutical agents that is outside of FDA-approved labelling. This information is intended solely for CME and is not intended to promote off-label use of these medications. If you have any questions, contact the medical affairs department of the manufacturer for the most recent prescribing information.

TO ENROLL

To enroll in the *Emergency Medicine Clinics* Continuing Medical Education program, call customer service at 1-800-654-2452 or sign up online at http://www.theclinics.com/home/cme. The CME program is available to subscribers for an additional annual fee of $212 USD.

METHOD OF PARTICIPATION

In order to claim credit, participants must complete the following:
1. Complete enrolment as indicated above.
2. Read the activity.
3. Complete the CME Test and Evaluation. Participants must achieve a score of 70% on the test. All CME Tests and Evaluations must be completed online.

CME INQUIRIES/SPECIAL NEEDS

For all CME inquiries or special needs, please contact elsevierCME@elsevier.com.

Foreword

Head, Eyes, Ears, Nose, and Throat Emergencies

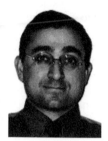

Amal Mattu, MD
Consulting Editor

During a recent survey of Emergency Department (ED) consulting practices in our medical center, I was shocked to discover which service our physicians had been consulting most frequently. It wasn't cardiology, neurology, critical care and not even general surgery. The service that was receiving the largest number of requests for ED consultations was oromaxillofacial (OMF) surgery. Not far behind in numbers of consultations was the ear, nose, and throat (ENT) service. I was surprised by this finding because most acute OMF and ENT emergencies don't strike me as life-threatening. They are not high-profile or well-publicized topics in journals or conferences, and they often tend to be triaged as more minor complaints. So why were we consulting the OMF and ENT services so frequently?

With a bit of further reflection, however, the answer became obvious. Frankly, many of us emergency physicians are not trained well in the management of these types of conditions. We spend far more of our time learning about and thinking about cardiovascular, neurologic, pulmonary, and gastrointestinal diseases. When it comes to the head, it seems that the main things we are interested in are the airway and the brain. Education regarding the teeth, the nose, the ear, the facial bones, and even the eyes tends to be relegated to a lower priority. A quick glance at any residency curriculum or conference brochure will confirm this. Yet, these "less exciting" parts of the body still account for a significant number of ED presentations. Even during my shift earlier today I saw a patient presenting with epistaxis, another patient with facial trauma that included a fracture and laceration, two patients with dental pain (including one that had a dental abscess), a patient transferred to us from a community hospital for the management of a peritonsillar abscess, and a patient with a sore throat (among other complaints). And yes, I did (sheepishly) consult the OMF and ENT services during the shift. If only I knew more about these conditions, I might have cared for the patients more quickly and spared the consultants some time.

Emerg Med Clin N Am 31 (2013) xi–xii
http://dx.doi.org/10.1016/j.emc.2013.03.002
0733-8627/13/$ – see front matter © 2013 Published by Elsevier Inc.

To our rescue come Drs Alisa Gibson and Kip Benko. These two physicians themselves are experts in OMF and ENT emergencies, having written and lectured about these topics nationally and internationally. As guest editors for this issue of *Emergency Medicine Clinics of North America*, they have assembled an outstanding group of authors to teach us much of what we should know but perhaps don't. The authors discuss facial fractures, dental pain and infections, epistaxis, ocular emergencies, and a host of other common emergencies pertaining to the head and face excluding the brain and airway. One additional article that I'm particularly thrilled to see pertains to the performance of regional nerve blocks of the face.

The guest editors and authors are to be commended for their hard work. This issue of *Emergency Medicine Clinics of North America* is an invaluable addition to the library of emergency physicians and other health care providers that care for acutely ill patients. More importantly, this is a must-read for students and residents training in emergency medicine. Drs Gibson, Benko, and colleagues have provided a comprehensive curriculum addressing the care of patients with OMF and ENT emergencies. The contributors are to be commended for providing this outstanding resource to us all.

Amal Mattu, MD
Department of Emergency Medicine
University of Maryland School of Medicine
Baltimore, MD 21201, USA

E-mail address:
amattu@smail.umaryland.edu

Preface

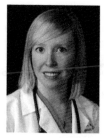 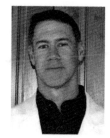

Alisa M. Gibson, MD, DMD   Kip R. Benko, MD, FACEP
Editors

Oropharyngeal and facial emergencies are commonly seen in Emergency Departments all over the country, whether suburban or rural. Presentations range from the relatively benign, such as dental pain, to life-threatening or vision-threatening conditions such as retrobulbar hematoma or massive hemorrhage. The emergency physician (EP) often has to address these complaints in the middle of the night, without any help from specialists. Rapid diagnosis and management are essential to permanent complications.

Orofacial complaints encompass a huge range of pathologic abnormality and specialty knowledge. Ophthalmologists, Otolaryngologists, Oral Maxillofacial Surgeons, and general dentists each spend years learning how to treat individual parts of facial and oropharyngeal structures, so it's understandable that complaints in these areas can often be anxiety provoking to the EP. This issue of *Emergency Medicine Clinics of North America* addresses the incredible scope of oropharyngeal and facial emergencies and hopefully serves to replace anxiety with confidence.

One of the challenges frequently facing the EP is which complaints must be addressed immediately versus which can be followed up by a specialist as an outpatient. Answers to that dilemma, along with pearls and pitfalls to improve patient outcomes and avoid disasters, are highlighted throughout the articles. We were fortunate to have outstanding authors contribute their substantial expertise and wisdom to these pages. We have certainly learned from them as we reviewed their work and are sure that you will as well.

We would like to thank the many individuals whose guidance and assistance made this project possible. We both have amazingly supportive and dedicated faculty and departmental leadership at our institutions, as well as stellar residents who constantly inspire and drive us to continue to learn and grow. We would also like to thank Amal

Emerg Med Clin N Am 31 (2013) xiii–xiv
http://dx.doi.org/10.1016/j.emc.2013.03.001
0733-8627/13/$ – see front matter © 2013 Published by Elsevier Inc.

emed.theclinics.com

Mattu for giving us this wonderful opportunity, and Patrick Manley for his support throughout the creation of this issue.

Alisa M. Gibson, MD, DMD
Department of Emergency Medicine
University of Maryland School of Medicine
110 South Paca Street, 6th Floor, Suite 200
Baltimore, MD 21201, USA

Kip R. Benko, MD, FACEP
Department of Emergency Medicine
University of Pittsburgh School of Medicine
Pittsburgh, PA, USA

E-mail addresses:
alisagibson@umem.org (A.M. Gibson)
kippster1@aol.com (K.R. Benko)

Ocular Inflammation and Infection

Jonathon P. Deibel, MD[a,b],*, Kathleen Cowling, DO, MS[a,b]

KEYWORDS

- Conjunctivitis • Hordeolum • Chalazion • Blepharitis • Scleritis • Episcleritis
- Keratitis • Iritis

KEY POINTS

- Blepharitis is treated with warm compresses and washes with mild soap; antibiotics should be considered for severe cases.
- Episcleritis is usually mild and self-limited; Scleritis can be severe and has an association with numerous systemic diseases.
- Chlamydia trachomatis presents initially as a watery discharge and progresses to a purulent discharge. Marked chemosis and eyelid swelling are present. Concurrent chlamydial pneumonia should be considered. Infected infants should be treated with oral erythromycin.
- Iritis presents with pain, blurred vision, and consensual photophobia. Concurrent systemic disease should be considered. Treatment consists of long-acting cycloplegics and oral analgesia.
- Corneal ulcers require frequent antibiotic dosing. Coverage of *Pseudomonas aeruginosa* should be provided to contact lens users. In addition to oral analgesics, a long-acting cycloplegic may provide some pain relief. Eye patching is not recommended for corneal abrasions or corneal ulcers.

Ocular inflammation and infection can occur in any part of the eye and surrounding tissue. The most common and most serious conditions seen in the emergency department are discussed here. It is important for an emergency physician to consider other sight-threatening conditions that can cause a painful acute red eye when considering the disposition and potential referral. Key signs and symptoms, common pathogens, and appropriate treatment and follow-up are discussed.

HORDEOLUM

A hordeolum (**Fig. 1**) is a pustular swelling of the lid margin, which is usually caused by *Staphylococcus aureus*. An internal hordeolum is a meibomian gland obstruction with

No funding support provided. No financial disclosures.

[a] Department of Emergency Medicine, Synergy Medical Education Alliance, 1000 Houghton Avenue, Saginaw, MI 48602, USA; [b] Michigan State University College of Human Medicine, 965 Fee Road, Room A-110, East Lansing, MI 48824, USA
* Corresponding author.
E-mail address: Jonathon.Deibel@cmich.edu

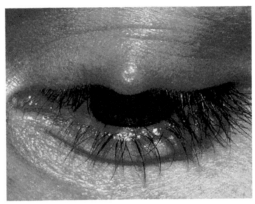

Fig. 1. Hordeolum. (*From* Seidel HM. Mosby's Guide to Physical Examination. Philadelphia: Elsevier Mosby, 2003; with permission.)

infection. An external hordeolum (synonymous with a sty) originates from a hair follicle or tear gland on the lid margin. Both forms usually resolve in about 1 week. Treatment consists of warm compresses. Although data on effectiveness are limited, antibiotic ophthalmic ointment may be considered. A hordeolum may develop into a chalazion and ultimately may require incision and drainage by an ophthalmologist.

CHALAZION

A chalazion is a nodular, granulomatous swelling of the eyelid caused by an obstruction of a meibomian gland or a gland of Zeis. It is usually not painful. The presentation is usually subacute or chronic, but it can be acute. A chalazion may develop from a hordeolum. Distinguishing the 2 may be impossible in the acute care setting. Treatment consists of warm compresses. Because a chalazion is often chronic, time to resolution is likely longer than with a hordeolum. Referral to an ophthalmologist for follow-up is appropriate, as steroid injection or incision and drainage may be indicated.

BLEPHARITIS

Blepharitis is chronic eyelid irritation and inflammation. Its cause is complex and still not entirely understood. Factors generally thought to contribute to this condition include microbial organisms (*S epidermidis* being primary), abnormal lid margin secretions, and abnormalities of the tear film.[1] Blepharitis has an association with atopic dermatitis, rosacea, and eczema.[2] Symptoms are multiple and varied, including irritation, tearing, pruritis, and flaking or crusting of the eyelid. The primary treatment of blepharitis is eyelid hygiene: warm massage with a moist washcloth about 20 minutes 4 times a day.[3] A cotton swab may be used with a mild baby shampoo to clean the lid margins twice a day. General consensus is in favor of topical or systemic antibiotics and topical steroids if the inflammation is severe.[1]

SCLERITIS AND EPISCLERITIS

Scleritis is inflammation of the sclera, whereas episcleritis is inflammation of the lining of the sclera, or episclera. Both have symptoms of blurred vision, photophobia, tearing, and severe pain, which tend to be worse at night. Episcleritis is usually mild and self-limited. Scleritis is often more severe and has a much higher association with systemic diseases such as Wegener granulomatosis, rheumatoid arthritis, and connective tissue disease. Scleritis also has a higher association with ocular complications, including uveitis, keratitis, ocular hypertension, and decrease in vision, potentially blindness.[4]

A diagnosis of idiopathic scleritis should prompt an investigation into systemic diseases. This evaluation should include urinalysis for protein and blood and serum testing of C-reactive protein, erythrocyte sedimentation rate, rheumatoid factor, antineutrophil cytoplasmic antibodies, and antinuclear antibodies levels.[5,6] Scleritis can be diffuse, nodular, or necrotizing. The diffuse pattern is the most common and benign form. Inflammation is widespread throughout the sclera. Nodular scleritis presents with one or more inflamed nodules on the sclera. Necrotizing scleritis has the highest association with systemic disease. It often presents with extreme pain and inflammation.

Treatment of scleritis depends on its severity.[7] Low severity, diffuse, or nodular scleritis responds best to oral nonsteroidal antiinflammatory drugs (NSAIDs). For high-severity scleritis, the use of topical steroidal antiinflammatory drugs (SAIDs) should be discussed with an ophthalmologist. Patients with accompanying systemic disease respond best to immunosuppressive therapy drugs or biologic response modifiers. Necrotizing scleritis responds best to immunosuppressive therapy drugs. Outpatient therapy is usually appropriate, together with prompt ophthalmology referral.

KERATITIS

Keratitis is inflammation of the cornea of the eye. It often induces intense pain. The primary causes are bacteria, viruses, and UV radiation. It also has fungal and amoebic sources. Exposure keratitis is caused by incomplete closure of the eyelid.

Bacterial causes of keratitis include *S aureus*, *Pseudomonas aeruginosa*, coagulase-negative staphylococci, diphtheroids, and *Streptococcus pneumonia*; polymicrobial infections have been reported as well.[8] Contact lens users are at increased risk for bacterial keratitis. *P aeruginosa* is the most common cause of bacterial keratitis in that group.[9] Symptoms include severe pain and a foreign body sensation. Examination may demonstrate a red eye, a corneal infiltrate, or an opacity that will stain with fluorescein. Hypopyon may be appreciated. Bacterial keratitis may also present with a mucopurulent discharge. Treatment includes topical antibiotics, oral analgesics, and prompt, same-day ophthalmology referral.

The most common cause of viral keratitis is herpes simplex virus (HSV). This diagnosis is based on the finding of branching or dendritic lesions revealed with fluorescein staining. Most cases of ophthalmic HSV infection are unilateral, but bilateral cases can occur in immunocompromised individuals.[10] The course of viral keratitis is ultimately self-limited; however, antiviral therapy is recommended because it shortens the duration of the infection.[11] The patient should see an ophthalmologist within a few days.

UV keratitis can be caused by sun exposure, skiing, welding, and germicidal UV lamps.[12] Patients present with severe pain that began 6 to 12 hours after exposure. Visual acuity may be decreased and eyes may be injected. There is generally no discharge from the eye as with infectious causes. A hazy, punctate staining is seen with fluorescein dye. Often a sharply demarcated affected zone is seen within the interpalpebral fissure from squinting at the time of exposure. Treatment consists of cycloplegic drops for pain relief and antibiotic drops or ointment for prophylaxis. Oral analgesics should be prescribed. Reevaluation within 2 or 3 days is appropriate.

DACRYOSTENOSIS

The nasolacrimal duct drains tears from the eye. An obstruction of this duct is known as dacryostenosis, which is very common in newborns and usually resolves spontaneously. This condition is not associated with erythema. Massage is first-line treatment. Continued obstruction may require probing by an ophthalmologist.

DACRYOCYSTOCELE

A dacryocystocele or dacryocele is a fluid collection in the nasolacrimal duct caused by blockage of the proximal or distal portions of the duct. Patients present with a bluish-gray mass at the medial canthus. Initial treatment is gentle digital massage. Ophthalmologic referral is required, as there is an association with intranasal polyps.

DACRYOCYSTITIS

Dacryocystitis (**Fig. 2**) is inflammation and swelling of the lacrimal sac from acute infection. The most common causative organisms include *S aureus, S pneumoniae, Haemophilus influenzae, Serratia marcescens*, and *P aeruginosa*.[13] In one study, 17.4% of cases of acute dacryocystitis were caused by *methicillin-resistant S aureus* (MRSA).[14] In infants, acute dacryocystitis represents a medical emergency, because it can lead to severe complications, including orbital cellulitis.[15] Cultures should be obtained by applying gentle pressure to the nasal lacrimal duct and expressing fluid. Treatment consists of massage, warm compresses, and systemic antibiotics. Antibiotic selection should include coverage of MRSA. Depending on the age of the patient and the acuity of the infection, probing or surgery may be required.

CELLULITIS

Cellulitis of the tissue surrounding the eye can be divided into periorbital and orbital categories (**Fig. 3**). Of the 2, a periorbital presentation is much more common. A distinction between them must be made, as orbital cellulitis can threaten both vision and life. Periorbital cellulitis is located anterior to the orbital septum. Orbital cellulitis is located posterior to the orbital septum but does not include the globe. The distinction can often be difficult and even impossible in the early stage of infection. Both forms may present with periorbital edema, fever, tearing, warmth, and erythema. A thorough examination may help to differentiate them. Generally there is no involvement of the eye with

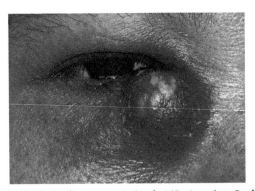

Fig. 2. Dacryocystitis. (*Courtesy of* Lawrence B. Stack, MD, Associate Professor of Emergency Medicine and Pediatrics Vanderbilt University Nashville, TN; with permission.)

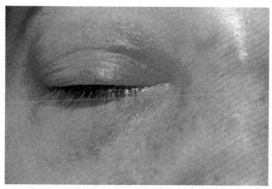

Fig. 3. Orbital cellulitis. (*From* CDC/Dr Thomas F. Sellers/Emory University. Public Health Image Library. Available at: http://phil.cdc.gov/.)

periorbital cellulitis. Proptosis, ophthalmoplegia, and pain with eye movement portend a diagnosis of orbital cellulitis or orbital abscess.[16] Sudden onset is also more likely with orbital cellulitis. A computed tomography (CT) scan or magnetic resonance imaging of the orbits is indicated in all cases of suspected orbital cellulitis. Orbital cellulitis has swelling posterior to the orbital septum on imaging. In straightforward cases of periorbital cellulitis, CT scanning is not necessary. An elevated white blood cell (WBC) count is more likely in association with orbital cellulitis; however, in up to 50% of adults, there is no elevation in this count.[17,18]

The most common cause of periorbital cellulitis is a contiguous facial infection such as sinusitis or hordeolum or an insect bite. Oral antibiotics and outpatient therapy are appropriate for mild cases of periorbital cellulitis in adults and nontoxic children. Appropriate antibiotic choice includes amoxicillin/clavulanate (Augmentin) or a first-generation cephalosporin. Prompt ophthalmology follow-up is recommended.

Most cases of orbital cellulitis are related to sinusitis.[19,20] Other causes include trauma, foreign body, dental infection, otitis media, and ophthalmic surgery.[21–23] Orbital cellulitis is often polymicrobial. Common pathogens include S aureus and streptococci.[24–26] Hospital admission, ophthalmology consultation, and intravenous (IV) antibiotics are indicated for all patients with confirmed or suspected orbital cellulitis. Antibiotics should cover both aerobic and anaerobic organisms. Appropriate antibiotic choices include ampicillin/sulbactam (Unasyn) or a first-generation cephalosporin in combination with metronidazole.[26] Complications include vision loss, subperiosteal abscess, orbital abscess, meningitis, osteomyelitis, and cavernous sinus thrombosis.[27]

CONJUNCTIVITIS

Conjunctivitis is a common cause of red eye presenting to the emergency department. The most common cause of conjunctivitis is infection. In children, bacterial conjunctivitis is more common than viral.[28] In adults, viral conjunctivitis is more common. Allergic, fungal, toxic, and chemical sources are also possible. Both viral and bacterial causes are highly infectious. Examination reveals injected bulbar conjunctiva. Other causes of red eye should be excluded before making the diagnosis of conjunctivitis. These include glaucoma, iritis, and keratitis. They can be ruled out by a detailed history, slit lamp examination, and measurement of intraocular pressure.

Bacterial conjunctivitis is usually painless and presents with copious purulent discharge. The likelihood of a bacterial cause is increased in patients who report having their eyes "stuck" closed in the morning and decreased with the complaint of pruritis.[29] The most common causes are *Streptococcus* and *Staphylococcus* species.[30] Recent studies found that 17% to 43% of cases of bacterial conjunctivitis are caused by MRSA and up to 21% are caused by *P aeruginosa*.[31–33] Fluorescein staining should be performed to avoid missing an ulcer, dendrite, or foreign body. Bacterial cultures are indicated in cases of severe or recurrent bacterial conjunctivitis and in all cases of neonatal conjunctivitis.[34] Although this condition is usually self-limited with clinical resolution in 2 to 5 days, patients with suspected and confirmed bacterial conjunctivitis should be treated with antibiotics because they reduce the time course and infectivity.[35–37] There are numerous choices for antibiotic therapy: erythromycin ophthalmic ointment, sulfacetamide ophthalmic (Bleph-10) drops, or polymyxin/trimethoprim (Polytrim) drops. For contact lens wearers, a fluoroquinolone or aminoglycoside is the best choice because *Pseudomonas* coverage is needed. For children, ointment is the better choice because it stays on the lid longer and continues to provide treatment. Drops may be preferred in adults, because the ointment temporarily blurs vision.

Two important causes of conjunctivitis are gonococcal and chlamydial (**Table 1**). Bacterial conjunctivitis caused by *Neisseria gonorrhoeae* is sight threatening. In neonates, it is called gonococcal ophthalmia neonatorum (**Fig. 4**). Its presentation is more pronounced than that of conjunctivitis of other causes. Patients have a hyperacute presentation of copious purulent discharge. The incubation period is 3 to 19 days. Concurrent urethritis may also be present. Gram stain shows gramnegative diplococci. Cultures are recommended in all cases of suspected *N gonorrhoeae* conjunctivitis. A single dose of IV or intramuscular ceftriaxone (Rocephin) is the recommended treatment.[38] Infants with gonococcal ophthalmia should be hospitalized for monitoring of possible disseminated infection, and both mother and infant should be tested for concurrent chlamydial infection.[38]

Chlamydial trachomatis in a newborn and young infant is of particular concern. Primary exposure is usually from the infected mother during vaginal childbirth. Presentation is usually between days 5 and 17 days of life.[39] Initially, a watery discharge is present. This discharge progresses to a purulent discharge, which is sometimes blood stained. The patient may have marked chemosis and eyelid swelling. Clinical suspicion of chlamydial conjunctivitis should prompt consideration for concurrent chlamydial pneumonia. Cultures should be performed in cases of suspected chlamydial conjunctivitis. Infants younger than 1 month of age, with a mother having a confirmed or suspected chlamydial infection or with concomitant pneumonia, are at increased risk for chlamydial conjunctivitis. The culture specimen should be taken from the

Table 1
Gonoccocal versus chlamydial conjunctivitis

	Gonococcal	Chlamydial
Presentation	Hyperacute; copious purulent discharge	Initial watery discharge; later purulent discharge; marked chemosis and eyelid swelling
Incubation	3–19 d	5–17 d
Treatment	IV or IM ceftriaxone	Oral erythromycin in infants; oral doxycycline or azithromycin in adults
Systemic complications	Meningitis, arthritis; septicemia	Pneumonia, otitis, reactive arthritis

Abbreviations: IM, intramuscular; IV, intravenous.

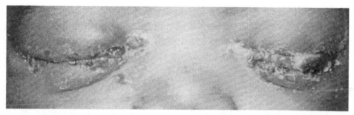

Fig. 4. Gonococcal ophthalmia neonatorum. (*From* CDC/J. Pledger. Public Health Image Library. Available at: http://phil.cdc.gov/.)

everted eyelid.[40] Oral erythromycin is the recommended treatment of infants with chlamydial conjunctivitis.[40,41]

Viral conjunctivitis presents with watery discharge. The patient may have conjunctival mucous, but no purulent discharge is present. Patients complain of irritation or a burning sensation. They may have other symptoms of a viral syndrome. Viral conjunctivitis is self-limited. Nonantibiotic lubricating drops may provide symptomatic relief, as may a topical antihistamine.[34]

Epidemic keratoconjunctivitis is an inflammation of the cornea and conjunctiva caused by a virus, usually an adenovirus. The virus is highly contagious and often presents in epidemics. The patient has typical viral conjunctivitis symptoms, but often much more severe. In addition, the patient has a foreign body sensation. Punctate keratitis can be appreciated on fluorescein staining. Currently, no effective drug therapy exists.[42] Treatment is directed toward symptoms (eg, artificial tears and cold compresses). Meticulous hygiene is of utmost importance in curtailing epidemics. Most cases spontaneously resolve in 1 to 3 weeks. In some cases, the corneal opacities seen initially as punctate keratitis may persist much longer. These can become vision threatening. Immediate referral to an ophthalmologist within 24 hours is required for surgery consideration and close monitoring.

Allergic conjunctivitis is caused by hypersensitivity to environmental or animal airborne allergens. The patient may have a history of seasonal or animal allergies. The primary complaint will be bilateral eye irritation, pruritis, and watery discharge. The patient often has chemosis. Antihistamine drops for symptom relief is the best treatment.

Nonallergic conjunctivitis is caused by dry eyes, trauma, a foreign body, or chemical irritation. It usually improves without intervention in 24 hours. Consider lubricant drops or ointment for treatment. The patient should be instructed against the use of over-the-counter vasoconstrictive drops, digital rubbing, and eye straining with reading.

IRITIS

Inflammation of the anterior portion of the uvea is known as iritis. Symptoms include pain, blurred vision, and consensual photophobia, which is pain in the affected eye when light is shined in the unaffected eye. The examination is significant for eye redness and may show a constricted, poorly reactive pupil. Slit lamp examination may show WBCs and flare in the anterior chamber. Fluorescein staining should be performed, as a corneal abrasion, foreign body, or ulceration might be present. Synechia (adhesion of the iris to the lens posteriorly or to the cornea anteriorly) may be seen in chronic disease. Iritis is usually unilateral, but it can be bilateral with systemic disease. Causes of iritis are multiple and should prompt consideration for systemic disease. Iritis may be caused by trauma, infection, malignancy, or inflammatory and autoimmune disorders. Silent disorders, such as syphilis, infection with the human immunodeficiency virus, and sarcoidosis, should be considered. Consider obtaining a chest film for sarcoidosis and serology testing for syphilis. Discomfort can be relieved with long-acting cycloplegics and oral analgesics. Prescription of an SAID should be discussed with an ophthalmologist. Consultation and prompt follow-up with an ophthalmologist is required.

HYPOPYON

A hypopyon occurs when exudate collects in the anterior chamber. It is seen as a yellow-white exudate that collects in the lower portion of the anterior chamber because of gravity when the patient is upright. A hypopyon is generally sterile, void of pathogens. The differential diagnosis includes iritis, corneal ulcer, endophthalmitis, and fungi. Treatment is directed at the cause.

CORNEAL ABRASION

A corneal abrasion is a defect to the corneal epithelium caused by trauma, foreign body injury, or contact lens use. Patients complain of severe pain and the sensation of a foreign body. Diagnosis is usually made by eliciting a history of trauma or a foreign body and confirmed with examination. Visual acuity may be normal. On examination, the pupil is typically found to be constricted due to reactive miosis. Fluorescein staining demonstrates an area of epithelial defect. Particular attention should be directed toward looking for Seidel sign, which is leaking of aqueous humor appreciated with staining. This sign indicates disruption of the globe, an ophthalmologic emergency. The lids should be everted to find and remove any foreign body. Treatment consists of antibiotic ointment for prophylaxis, lubrication, and narcotic analgesia. Topical NSAIDs also provide some symptomatic relief. A cycloplegic may be used to prevent reactive cyclospasm, especially if the lesion involves the visual center of the cornea. Eye patching is not recommended because it provides no additional pain relief or acceleration of healing.[43,44] Limited data suggest tetanus prophylaxis is appropriate only in cases of globe perforation and infection but not in cases of superficial corneal abrasion; however, the current practice of emergency physicians is variable, with a tendency toward giving the tetanus vaccine.[45,46]

CORNEAL ULCER

A corneal ulcer is caused by a break in the epithelium of the cornea, initiated by trauma or an infection. Patients have pain, tearing, photophobia, and a foreign body sensation. *Staphylococcus* and *Streptococcus* species are the most common pathogens in noncontact lens wearers. In contact lens wearers, *Pseudomonas* and fungi are common pathogens.[47] Ulcers are more common in people who wear contact lenses, specifically soft contact lenses. Review of the patient's medication history may reveal the use of immunosuppressant agents including steroids. Examination reveals a whitish corneal infiltrate, which is better visualized with fluorescein dye. The patient may also have lid edema and conjunctival hyperemia. Topical antibiotics should be initiated. A fluoroquinolone is a good choice, because it provides excellent *Pseudomonas* coverage. A fortified antibiotic drop consisting of an aminoglycoside and a first-generation cephalosporin can also be chosen. Corneal ulcers require much more frequent application of antibiotic drops than needed for other ophthalmologic infections. A long-acting cycloplegic may be considered for relaxation of associated ciliary muscle spasm, which can contribute significantly to the patient's pain. Ophthalmology consultation and follow-up within 24 hours is required.

SUMMARY

Ocular inflammation and infection may involve any part of the eye and surrounding tissue. A complete examination, including visual acuity, extraocular movements, pupillary response, intraocular pressure, slit lamp examination, and fluorescein staining, is often required to establish the diagnosis. Adequate pain relief may be achieved with oral analgesics and cycloplegics. Topical anesthetic drops should not be prescribed. Patients should be advised to avoid rubbing their eyes or straining them with excessive reading. In most cases, prompt follow-up is required because vision loss may be a possibility.

ACKNOWLEDGEMENTS

This manuscript was copyedited by Linda J. Kesselring, MS, ELS, the technical editor/writer in the Department of Emergency Medicine at the University of Maryland School of Medicine.

REFERENCES

1. Jackson WB. Blepharitis: current strategies for diagnosis and management. Can J Ophthalmol 2008;43:170–9.
2. Driver PJ, Lemp MA. Meibomian gland dysfunction. Surv Ophthalmol 1996;40(5): 343–67.
3. Gilbard JP. The diagnosis and management of dry eyes. Otolaryngol Clin North Am 2005;38:871–85.
4. Sainz de la Maza M, Molina N, Gonzalez-Gonzalez LA, et al. Clinical characteristics of a large cohort of patients with scleritis and episcleritis. Ophthalmology 2012;119(1):43–50.
5. Lin P, Bhullar SS, Tessler HH, et al. Immunologic markers as potential predictors of systemic autoimmune disease in patients with idiopathic scleritis. Am J Ophthalmol 2008;145(3):463–71.
6. Hoang LT, Lim LL, Vaillant B, et al. Antineutrophil cytoplasmic antibody-associated active scleritis. Arch Ophthalmol 2008;126(5):651–5.
7. Sainz de la Maza M, Molina N, Gonzalez-Gonzalez LA, et al. Scleritis therapy. Ophthalmology 2012;119(1):51–8.
8. Hindman HB, Patel SB, Jun AS. Rationale for adjunctive topical corticosteroids in bacterial keratitis. Arch Ophthalmol 2009;127:97–102.
9. Stapleton F, Carnt N. Contact lens-related microbial keratitis: how have epidemiology and genetics helped us with pathogenesis and prophylaxis. Eye (Lond) 2012;26(2):185–93.
10. Souza PM, Holland EJ, Huang AJ. Bilateral herpetic keratoconjunctivitis. Ophthalmology 2003;110(3):493–6.
11. Wilhelmus KR. Therapeutic interventions for herpes simplex virus epithelial keratitis. Cochrane Database Syst Rev 2008;(1):CD002898.
12. Banerjee S, Patwardhan A, Savant VV. Mass photokeratitis following exposure to unprotected ultraviolet light. J Public Health Med 2003;25:160.
13. Pinar-Sueiro S, Fernández-Hermida RV, Gibelalde A, et al. Study on the effectiveness of antibiotic prophylaxis in external dacryocystorhinostomy: a review of 697 cases. Ophthal Plast Reconstr Surg 2010;26(6):467–72.
14. Mills D, Bodman MG, Meyer DR, et al. The microbiologic spectrum of dacryocystitis: a national study of acute versus chronic infection. Ophthal Plast Reconstr Surg 2007;23:302–6.

15. Campolattaro BN, Lueder GT, Tychsen L. Spectrum of pediatric dacryocystitis: medical and surgical management of 54 cases. J Pediatr Ophthalmol Strabismus 1997;34:143–53.
16. Rudloe TF, Harper MB, Prabhu SP. Acute periorbital infections: who needs emergent imaging? Pediatrics 2010;125(4):e719–26.
17. Weiss A, Friendly D, Eligin K, et al. Bacterial periorbital and orbital cellulitis in children. Ophthalmology 1983;90:195–203.
18. Robinson A, Beech T, McDermott AL, et al. Investigation and management of adult periorbital and orbital cellulitis. J Laryngol Otol 2006;121:545–7.
19. Ambati BK, Ambati J, Azar N, et al. Periorbital and orbital cellulitis before and after the advent of Haemophilus influenzae type B vaccination. Ophthalmology 2000;107:1450–3.
20. DeMuri GP, Wald ER. Complications of acute bacterial sinusitis in children. Pediatr Infect Dis J 2011;30(8):701–2.
21. Weakley DR. Orbital cellulitis complicating strabismus surgery: a case report and review of the literature. Ann Ophthalmol 1991;23(12):454–7.
22. Allan BP, Egbert MA, Myall RW. Orbital abscess of odontogenic origin: case report and review of the literature. Int J Oral Maxillofac Surg 1991;20(5):268–70.
23. Rubinstein JB, Handler SD. Orbital and periorbital cellulitis in children. Head Neck Surg 1982;5(1):15–21.
24. Seltz LB, Smith J, Durairaj VD, et al. Microbiology and antibiotic management of orbital cellulitis. Pediatrics 2011;127(3):e566–72.
25. McKinley SH, Yen MT, Miller AM, et al. Microbiology of pediatric orbital cellulitis. Am J Ophthalmol 2007;144(4):497–501.
26. Nageswaran S, Woods CR, Benjamin DK Jr, et al. Orbital cellulitis in children. Pediatr Infect Dis J 2006;25(8):695–9.
27. Chaudhry IA, Shamsi FA, Elzaridi E, et al. Outcome of treated orbital cellulitis in a tertiary eye care center in the middle East. Ophthalmology 2007;114: 345–54.
28. Weiss A, Brinser JH, Nazar-Stewart V. Acute conjunctivitis in childhood. J Pediatr 1993;122:10–4.
29. Rietveld RP, ter Riet G, Bindels PJ, et al. Predicting bacterial cause in infectious conjunctivitis: cohort study on informativeness of combinations of signs and symptoms. BMJ 2004;329:206–10.
30. Friedlaender MH. A review of the causes and treatment of bacterial and allergic conjunctivitis. Clin Ther 1995;17:800–10.
31. Cavuoto K, Zytshi D, Karp C, et al. Update on bacterial conjunctivitis in South Florida. Ophthalmology 2008;115:51–6.
32. Asbell PA, Colby KA, Deng S, et al. Ocular TRUST: nationwide antimicrobial susceptibility patterns in ocular isolates. Am J Ophthalmol 2008;145:951–8.
33. Adebayo A, Parikh JG, McCormick SA, et al. Shifting trends in in vitro antibiotic susceptibilities for common bacterial conjunctival isolates in the last decade at the New York Eye and Ear Infirmary. Graefes Arch Clin Exp Ophthalmol 2011; 249:111–9.
34. American Academy of Opthalmology Cornea/External Disease Panel. Preferred Practice Pattern Guidelines. Conjunctivitis - Limited Revision. San Francisco (CA): American Academy of Opthalmology; 2011. Available at: www.aao.org/ppp.
35. Sheikh A, Hurwitz B. Antibiotics versus placebo for acute bacterial conjunctivitis. Cochrane Database Syst Rev 2006;(2):CD001211.
36. Sheikh A, Hurwitz B. Topical antibiotics for acute bacterial conjunctivitis: a systematic review. Br J Gen Pract 2001;51:473–7.

37. Epling J. Bacterial conjunctivitis. Clin Evid 2012. pii:0704.
38. Centers for Disease Control and Prevention. Sexually Transmitted Disease Treatment Guidlines 2010. MMWR 2012;59(no. RR-12): 51, 54.
39. Remington JS, Klein JO, Wilson CB, et al. Infectious disease of the fetus and newborn. 7th edition. Philadelphia: Elsevier Saunders; 2010. p. 600.
40. Workowski KA, Berman S, Centers for Disease Control and Prevention (CDC). Sexually transmitted diseases treatment guidelines, 2010. MMWR Recomm Rep 2010;59:1–110.
41. American Academy of Pediatrics. Chlamydia trachomatis. In: Pickering LK, editor. Red book: 2009 report of the committee on infectious diseases. 28th edition. Elk Grove Village (IL): American Academy of Pediatrics; 2009. p. 255–9.
42. Meyer-Rüsenberg B, Loderstädt U, Richard G, et al. Epidemic keratoconjunctivitis: the current situation and recommendations for prevention and treatment. Dtsch Arztebl Int 2011;108(27):475–80.
43. Arbour JD, Brunette I, Boisjoly HM, et al. Should we patch corneal erosions? Arch Ophthalmol 1997;115:313–7.
44. Fraser S. Corneal abrasion. Clin Ophthalmol 2010;4:387–90.
45. Mukherjee P, Sivakumar A. Tetanus prophylaxis in superficial corneal abrasions. Emerg Med J 2003;20(1):62–4.
46. Calder L, Balasubramanian S, Stiell I. Lack of consensus on corneal abrasion management: results of a national survey. CJEM 2004;6(6):402–7.
47. Jeng BH, Gritz DC, Kumar AB, et al. Epidemiology of ulcerative keratitis in Northern California. Arch Ophthalmol 2010;128(8):1022–8.

Ocular Trauma and Other Catastrophes

Victoria M. Romaniuk, MD

KEYWORDS

- Hyphema • Globe rupture • Retrobulbar hemorrhage • Angle closure glaucoma
- Retinal detachment • Eye trauma

KEY POINTS

- Twenty-five percent of traumatic open-globe injuries are associated with orbital and adnexal injuries.
- Computed tomography cannot be relied on alone to diagnose globe rupture; in patients with high suspicion, formal surgical exploration is the standard of care.
- In the setting of open-globe injuries, an intraocular foreign body is present up to 41% of the time and should be strongly considered in penetrating globe injuries.
- In the setting of retrobulbar hemorrhage with orbital compartment syndrome, decompression must occur within 90 minutes after injury to reduce the risk of vision loss.
- Penetrating injury to the posterior segment can cause acute retinal detachment, whereas blunt injury typically causes delayed retinal detachment.
- The combination of new-onset floaters and flashing lights should be considered retinal detachment until proved otherwise.

More than 1 million people worldwide have lost vision in both eyes as a result of trauma. In addition, unilateral blinding injuries have an incidence of 500,000 cases, making trauma one of the leading causes of unilateral blindness.[1] Traumatic ocular complaints account for 3% of emergency department (ED) visits in the United States. Ocular injuries range from simple abrasions to devastating globe ruptures. Regardless of mechanism, all injuries can result in some degree of vision loss, whether acutely or delayed. It is necessary for the emergency physician to be aware of emergent management options that can restore vision, whether related to trauma or some other catastrophe. The initiation of emergent measures can reduce complications while awaiting definitive specialty management.

GLOBE RUPTURE

Open-globe injuries refer to the presence of full-thickness scleral or corneal wounds, resulting from either blunt force (globe rupture) or penetrating or lacerating mechanisms

Department of Emergency Medicine, University of Maryland School of Medicine, 6th Floor, Suite 200, 110 South Paca Street, Baltimore, MD 21201, USA
E-mail address: vromaniuk@umem.org

Emerg Med Clin N Am 31 (2013) 399–411
http://dx.doi.org/10.1016/j.emc.2013.02.003
0733-8627/13/$ – see front matter © 2013 Elsevier Inc. All rights reserved.

emed.theclinics.com

of injury (which include the introduction of an intraocular foreign body).[1] Globe ruptures usually occur on the anterior surface of the eye (where the sclera is thinnest), allowing the protrusion of intraocular structures or contents to be readily evident. When the rupture occurs posteriorly (occult) little damage is visible anteriorly, so the provider must have a high level of suspicion for this injury. Clinical findings suggestive of occult rupture include a shallow anterior chamber and decreased intraocular pressure (IOP), especially compared with the opposite eye.[2] Additional findings suggesting globe rupture include bullous 360° bulbar subconjunctival hemorrhage, limited extraocular motility, peaked or irregular pupil, or lens material in the anterior chamber.[3] On slit-lamp examination, when open-globe injury is not certain, fluorescein drops applied to the eye can allow visualization of aqueous fluid leaking from a wound when the cobalt blue light is illuminated (Seidel sign), indicating a full-thickness injury.

When examining a patient with any trauma to the face and orbit, always consider globe rupture. A detailed history is essential for assessment and consideration of globe rupture, specifically regarding the circumstance and mechanism of injury. Timing of injury and onset of symptoms should be documented.

If rupture is obvious, further examination should be deferred to an ophthalmologist, which will often occur in the operating room.[4] In addition, application of pressure to the eye must be avoided, as this may further expel intraocular contents.[1] Evaluation of the patient must include assessment of visual acuity (which can indicate prognostic outcomes), pupil reactivity (afferent pupillary defect indicates posterior injury), ocular motility, and slit-lamp examination.

The emergency physician is responsible for the identification and management of concomitant injuries. Given the high force of energy needed to cause globe rupture, the patient is likely to have associated facial and orbital injuries. In a retrospective chart review of 300 patients with traumatic open-globe injuries resulting from both blunt and penetrating mechanisms, Hatton and colleagues[5] found that 25% were associated with orbital and adnexal injuries. The most common associated injuries were periocular lacerations, orbital fracture, and retrobulbar hemorrhage. Patients with globe rupture and associated extraocular injuries presented with worse visual acuity than those without associated injuries.

Imaging can be performed to assess concomitant injuries and foreign bodies, and, in most cases, to assist in diagnosing globe rupture. The sensitivity of computed tomography (CT) for identifying occult open-globe injuries has been reported to be 56% to 75%, with specificity ranging from 76% to 100%.[4] Therefore, CT cannot be relied on alone for diagnosis of globe rupture. When suspicion for this injury is high, formal surgical exploration is the standard of care. CT findings suggestive of open-globe injury include intraocular air, change in globe contour, and scleral discontinuity (**Fig. 1**). Ocular ultrasonography has also been useful in the evaluation of ocular injury but is contraindicated in patients with globe rupture, who should be referred to an ophthalmologist.

ED management of patients with globe rupture consists of emergent ophthalmology consultation for immediate surgical repair. Additional measures include assessment of tetanus status, placement of a rigid ocular shield, administration of systemic analgesia and antiemetics, elevation of the head of bed, and administration of systemic antibiotics to reduce the risk of endophthalmitis.[1,3] The occurrence of endophthalmitis following open-globe injury ranges from 2.6% to 30%, with cultured organisms such as staphylococci, streptococci, and bacilli.[6] Based on these findings, despite a lack of randomized clinical trials, administration of prophylactic empiric systemic antibiotics in the setting of open globe injury is the standard of care. The recommended antibiotics are cefazolin or vancomycin and a fourth-generation fluoroquinolone.

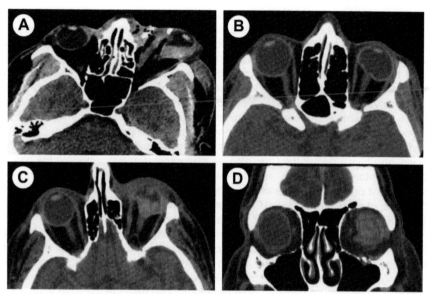

Fig. 1. Globe rupture. Open-globe injury. Axial CT (*A*) shows posterior rupture of the left globe with vitreous hemorrhage. Note the conical globe deformity. (*B*) Axial CT from another patient with posterior globe rupture demonstrates a flattened irregular contour: the "flattened tire" sign. Axial (*C*) and coronal (*D*) images from a third patient illustrate the heterogeneous appearance of intraocular hemorrhage, with a ruptured and deformed posterior globe associated with a subluxed lens following trauma. (*From* Dunkin JM, Crum AV, Swanger R, et al. The globe trauma. Semin Ultrasound CT MR 2011;32(1):51–6; with permission.)

In the series reported by Al-Mezaine and colleagues,[7] good visual outcomes after surgical management were achieved in patients who presented with visual acuity of 20/200 or better, age 18 years or younger, sharp injuries (opposed to blunt), anterior wound location (opposed to posterior), and absence of associated ocular injuries. Poor visual outcomes in patients with open-globe injuries include afferent pupillary defect, lens damage, and the presence of an intraocular foreign body.[5]

FOREIGN BODIES

Evaluation of ocular foreign bodies can be challenging in the ED. The diagnosis is often suggested by the history provided by the patient, with special attention to the circumstances under which the symptoms emerged. Ocular foreign bodies can be superficial, embedded in the conjunctiva or cornea, or intraocular. Intraocular foreign bodies (IOFBs) are present in 10.2% of patients with ocular injuries.[8] IOFBs can present dramatically but often are subtle. Multiple foreign bodies might be present. An undetected or undiagnosed IOFB can lead to vision-threatening complications. The United Eye Injury Registry has found that 25% of patients who sustain an IOFB injury have poor final visual acuity, less than 20/200.[9] Therefore, it is the responsibility of the ED physician to identify the location and composition of ocular foreign bodies, either superficial or intraocular, and remove those that are superficial. However, as with all eye trauma, more serious, life-threatening injuries should be stabilized before evaluation of the globe.

The history of the injurious event should be ascertained, with attention to the mechanism (eg, explosive device, tree branch, shattered glass), the velocity, and the timing of injury. These factors can help determine the location of a foreign body, be it superficial, intraocular, or both. Activities and events with a high risk of IOFBs include the use of power tools, the discharge of projectile weapons (guns, BB guns), motor vehicle crashes, metal-on-metal impacts, and any high-impact trauma.[9,10] The most common ocular foreign body is metal, often resulting from the mechanism of hammering. A patient who reports this activity in his or her history might have a high-velocity penetrating injury and is likely to have a metallic foreign body.[11,12] IOFBs are present in up to 41% of patients with open-globe injuries, and therefore should be strongly considered when assessing patients with penetrating globe injuries.[13]

Symptoms of superficial foreign bodies include eye pain, foreign body sensation, tearing, and blurry vision; they can also be asymptomatic, suggested by the history alone. Symptoms suggestive of intraocular penetration can be minimal, and the patient might present only after complications arise. The ED physician must maintain a high level of suspicion of IOFB if the history (such as occupation) and clinical presentation are suggestive, regardless of the patient's symptoms.

When evaluating a patient with symptoms suggesting an IOFB, first perform a gross inspection to assess for signs of open-globe injury, such as prolapsed intraocular structures, an irregularly shaped (often peaked) pupil, or intraocular contents prolapsing from the eye. If open-globe injury is obvious, further manipulation of the globe should be deferred until an ophthalmologist can manage the case in an operating room.

Note the patient's visual acuity and perform a slit-lamp examination without and with fluorescein. Document the size, depth, and location of corneal foreign bodies. Signs of deep injuries include inflammation or hemorrhage of the anterior chamber, corneal or scleral wounds, iris transillumination, and lens opacities. The presence of corneal infiltrate or hypopion indicates infection, and its detection should prompt referral to an ophthalmologist. If it is not clear if an open-globe injury is present, perform the Seidel test to assess for leakage of aqueous fluid. The examination can be facilitated by the application of a topical anesthetic. Perform a fundoscopic examination early to assess for the presence of an IOFB, because visualization of the posterior segment can be difficult once vitreous hemorrhage, corneal edema, or cataract develops in response to an IOFB.[9,10] In a limited retrospective case review, the finding of IOFB on fundoscopic examination in patients with a corneal metal foreign body without clinical evidence of penetrating injury was very rare.[14]

After applying a topical anesthetic, remove small, loose conjunctival foreign bodies with copious irrigation or with the edge of a cotton-tipped swab soaked in saline.[15] Evert the lids to evaluate their underside for embedded subtarsal foreign bodies, which are often suggested by the presence of linear corneal abrasions. Corneal foreign bodies can be removed under visualization with a slit lamp and the use of a 30- to 25-gauge needle if irrigation is not successful. The presence of a full-thickness corneal foreign body is considered an open-globe injury and should be managed by an ophthalmologist. If attempted removal of a foreign body is unsuccessful or if the patient is uncooperative, defer management to an ophthalmologist urgently. Rust rings indicate the presence of an iron-containing foreign body. If a rust ring is present, an ophthalmic burr can be used to remove the superficial rust, with repeat evaluation and further management within 24 hours by an ophthalmologist. It is important that the ED physician should not attempt to remove rust rings that are deep or embedded in the visual axis (pupil), because of the risk of scarring and visual impairment.[16]

Imaging studies can facilitate further assessment of IOFBs. Plain films, though easy to obtain, detect only about 40% of IOFB[9,10,17] and therefore are not usually obtained for this purpose. Most useful are CT scans, which have sensitivities reaching 95%.[8] CT imaging is most useful for detection of metal, glass, and stone.[4] Adesanya and Dawkins[18] reported a case in which intraocular wood was seen as intraorbital air on CT imaging; this possibility can be considered when air is seen in the absence of fracture. Magnetic resonance imaging can facilitate visualization of IOFBs that are radiolucent on CT scan, but its use is limited because the presence of metal is a contraindication. Therefore, when a CT scan does not identify metal or any foreign body, MRI can be used when wooden or vegetative foreign bodies are suspected.[19] Ultrasonography is able to detect IOFBs, but its use is limited to experienced technicians and should not be performed in the setting of open-globe injury.

Iron, copper, lead, zinc, and nickel can cause toxicity to ocular structures and launch an inflammatory response that can lead to irreversible vision loss.[9,10] The presence of these materials should prompt emergent ophthalmology referral.

Management of superficial foreign bodies includes their removal from the conjunctiva or cornea, as previously discussed. Subsequently, the eye should be irrigated copiously and the Seidel sign reaffirmed to indicate that removal did not perforate the cornea. Although further management is lacking in clinical controlled trials, recommendations include systemic analgesics as needed, tetanus booster as warranted, cycloplegics for discomfort, and prophylactic topical antibiotics for corneal involvement.[20] Topical antibiotics should be aimed at covering gram-positive organisms, with the addition of *Pseudomonas* coverage in contact-lens wearers. Follow-up with an ophthalmologist can be scheduled on an outpatient basis for uncomplicated presentations.

Management of IOFBs includes systemic analgesia, antiemetics, and tetanus booster if necessary, prophylactic empiric antibiotics to protect against endophthalmitis, placement of a rigid eye shield, and emergent ophthalmology management. The incidence of endophthalmitis after IOFB ranges from 1.3% to 60%.[9,10] Retrospective studies have shown that gram-positive organisms, with few gram-negative and fungal organisms identified, cause the majority of cases of posttraumatic endophthalmitis. Although there are multiple recommendations, there is little evidence indicating that the use of prophylactic antibiotics, or a specific combination of such, is appropriate. Administration of systemic fluoroquinolone has been suggested in most cases for broad-spectrum coverage and vitreal penetration.[11,21] The use of antibiotics can be discussed in consultation with an ophthalmologist.

RETROBULBAR HEMATOMA

Retrobulbar hematoma (RBH), also known as retrobulbar hemorrhage, is a rare but vision-threatening emergency. Bleeding into the retrobulbar space within the confined walls of the orbit can increase IOP. This pressure can be transmitted to the optic nerve and globe, resulting in compression of retinal vessels, causing retinal ischemia.[13] The resultant loss of vision is irreversible within 60 to 100 minutes after the onset of ischemia.[1,22] McClenaghan and colleagues[23] and Shek and colleagues[24] described this condition secondary to trauma as traumatic orbital compartment syndrome (OCS). In OCS, additional optic nerve damage is caused by retrobulbar edema compressing the optic nerve vasculature and optic nerve directly. RBH can occur after blunt or penetrating facial trauma, orbital surgery, endoscopic sinus surgery, and retrobulbar injections, or even spontaneously. The incidence of retrobulbar hemorrhage from zygomatic complex facial fractures is 0.3%.[23] Traumatic RBH typically involves arterial bleeding, specifically from rupture of the infraorbital artery or ethmoidal arteries.[25,26]

Displaced fractures of the orbital bones tend to allow blood to evacuate from the orbit, and so are less likely to result in OCS. However, Popat and colleagues[25] treated a 77-year-old woman who had an orbital floor fracture but still developed RBH, which led to OCS and permanent vision loss.

Traumatic RBH can develop within a few hours after injury or much later. Ghufoor and colleagues[27] described a patient who had delayed onset of retrobulbar hemorrhage, 7 days after severe head injury. In cases such as this other diagnoses must be considered, such as orbital cellulitis or abscess, cavernous sinus thrombosis, orbital emphysema, and fistula.

RBH with OCS is usually diagnosed based on clinical signs and symptoms, and treatment must not be delayed for imaging studies unless a life-threatening injury is considered, such as intracranial hemorrhage. In addition, given the likelihood of concomitant injuries, most life-threatening injuries, such as airway compromise, should be addressed first. Clinical signs strongly suggesting RBH with OCS include the presence of 3 or more of the following: pain, decreased vision, proptosis with resistance to retropulsion, chemosis, limited extraocular motility, diplopia, diffuse subconjunctival hemorrhage, increased IOP, and afferent pupillary defect.[23] Development of OCS is a dynamic process, and these features may not be present on arrival in the ED; therefore, serial examinations should be performed to evaluate the patient for progression of symptoms. Fundoscopy may reveal edema of the optic disc, retinal edema, or retinal venous congestion.[28]

Once the diagnosis is established, the orbit must be decompressed immediately to restore vision. Several studies suggest that delayed treatment of OCS will likely result in permanent loss of vision.[28] Medical treatments, lateral canthotomy, and inferior cantholysis should be initiated in the ED, ideally within 90 minutes after injury.[25] However, even if the injury is thought to have occurred hours or days ago, there is no way to determine when the suspected RBH reached the critical pressure that caused vision loss. Lima and colleagues[28] observed that 12 of 16 patients with RBH and OCS recovered vision, with decompression occurring within a mean of 30 hours after onset of symptoms. ED management will only "buy time" until definitive surgical management is performed, so ophthalmology consultation and referral must be arranged immediately, whether or not emergent canthotomy is performed.[1] Despite decompression of high intraorbital pressure with lateral canthotomy and inferior cantholysis, typically only a small amount of blood is expressed.[22] Vision may improve dramatically within the first 15 minutes, but this process can also take up to 6 months, depending on the timing of decompression in relation to the onset of injury.[3]

Medical management has been shown to be effective in visual outcomes,[23,25] and can be initiated concomitantly with lateral canthotomy. Pharmacologic management aims to reduce IOP, which can be achieved with carbonic anhydrase inhibitors and hyperosmotic fluid. Additional measures to reduce IOP should be instituted, including elevation of the head, applying ice packs to the orbits, and administration of systemic analgesia and antiemetics.[3,25]

When the diagnosis is uncertain or if initial decompression fails to relieve OCS, imaging studies can be performed with CT scan or ocular ultrasonography. Findings on CT scan indicative of RBH include severe proptosis and tented posterior sclera with stretching of the optic nerve.[1] Rarely is a discrete hematoma identified on a CT scan.[3] CT offers the advantage of identifying additional injuries frequently associated with RBH: orbital and facial fractures, intraocular foreign body, penetrating facial injuries, and intracranial injuries. Bedside ocular ultrasonography identifies RBH as lucency deep to the retina and anterior to the orbit.[29] Although this can help to quickly establish the diagnosis of RBH, the absence of findings on a sonogram may not be sufficient in a patient who is at risk of developing RBH. For these patients, observation for at least 12 hours is recommended for serial ocular examinations.[3]

In the absence of trauma, spontaneous RBH must be considered in patients who have or are at risk of venous anomalies or bleeding disorders. In a retrospective study of 115 cases of nontraumatic RBH, Sullivan and Wright[30] found that 97 were due to venous anomalies and 4 to coagulopathies. These conditions should be considered and investigations undertaken to manage underlying causes.

HYPHEMA

Blunt or penetrating trauma to the orbit can result in vessel disruption of the ciliary body and iris, leading to collection of blood in the anterior chamber, known as hyphema.[9] This condition alone uncommonly leads to permanent loss of vision, but its presence can indicate the possibility of other acute vision-threatening injuries, such as globe rupture. In urban medical centers, about 60% of traumatic hyphemas result from blunt trauma, whereas about 30% result from penetrating trauma.[31] The peak incidence occurs in people between the ages 10 and 20 years, with an average age of less than 25 years.[31]

Patients who sustain traumatic hyphemas may complain of pain and impaired vision. The initial assessment of a patient with blunt or penetrating injury to the face or globe should consist of a full and detailed history. Specifically, the following information should be ascertained: the mechanism of injury (force, velocity, type), time of injury, timing of onset of symptoms, use of protective eyewear, use of medications (anticoagulants, antiplatelets), history of coagulopathy or bleeding diathesis, and personal or family history of sickle-cell trait or anemia.[2] Patients with sickle-cell trait or anemia have a higher incidence of complications following hyphema.[32] Ocular examination should consist of evaluation for other traumatic injuries, specifically addressing possible globe or scleral rupture. Eighty-three percent of patients with traumatic hyphema sustain more than 1 structural injury, with corneal abrasions being the most common (26%–40%).[32] CT scan can be considered to evaluate for concomitant injuries, but is not useful for the identification of hyphema. Evaluation of the adnexa, assessment of visual acuity and ocular motility, and a fundoscopic examination should be performed to assess for other ocular injuries. Abnormal pupillary response, such as Marcus Gunn pupil, indicates posterior segment or optic nerve injury. Signs of hyphema can be seen best on slit-lamp examination, with the patient sitting upright, as red blood cell sediment in the anterior chamber. The sediment typically separates into layers with a "fluid level," the height of which should be measured and documented on initial assessment.[2] This measurement will be useful to assess for subsequent active bleeding or secondary hemorrhage. Hyphemas are classified from grade 1 to grade 4, based on the volume of red blood cells identified. Microhyphema refers to the presence of circulating red blood cells that do not layer in the anterior chamber, whereas grade 4 refers to total or "8-ball" hyphema, in which the entire anterior chamber is filled with blood.[32]

Approximately one-third of all hyphema patients have increased IOP.[31] The pressure should be measured, unless evidence suggests globe rupture. If it is suspected that the globe might have ruptured, no pressure should be applied to it, so as to avoid additional trauma. The degree of IOP is not necessarily directly proportional to the size of the hyphema, although it is generally observed that the larger the hyphema volume, the greater likelihood of increased IOP. Therefore, in the setting of total hyphema, a measured IOP that is normal or low may raise concern for ruptured globe.[31]

A plan for definitive management should be designed in consultation with an ophthalmologist. ED management should consist of a thorough evaluation for and management of additional injuries (such as ruptured globe, facial fractures, corneal abrasions, intraocular foreign bodies), and management of elevated IOP. In the setting of increased IOP (>30 mm Hg), medical therapy should be aimed at lowering the pressure, with the goal of reducing vision loss. This treatment consists of the topical application of β-blockers and oral or intravenous administration of carbonic anhydrase inhibitors, such as acetazolamide, and/or hyperosmotic fluid, such as mannitol. Special consideration must be given to systemic diseases that would contraindicate such interventions. Specifically, sickle-cell trait or anemia would limit use of acetazolamide, because the resultant metabolic acidosis would induce sickling of blood cells within the anterior chamber and further elevate IOP. Therefore, methazolamide would be preferred in this patient population.[32]

Complications of hyphema include secondary bleeding (rebleeding), corneal blood staining, anterior synechiae, optic atrophy, and glaucoma. Such complications are even worse in the setting of rebleeding, which occurs within 1 to 7 days in up to 33% of patients with hyphema.[9] It has been suggested that rebleeding occurs secondary to clot lysis and retraction. Therefore, aspirin should be avoided or discontinued in patients with hyphema.

Additional therapy initiated with specialty consultation is aimed at prevention of complications, such as rebleeding and prolonged periods of elevated IOP.[9] Based on a literature review and meta-analysis, Gharaibeh and colleagues[33] concluded that antifibrinolytics, such as aminocaproic acid, can reduce the rate of secondary bleeding but can have other side effects such as nausea and vomiting. The use of these agents should be weighed against potential complications, as additional studies show that they are of no statistical benefit. The individual consulting ophthalmologist should select additional measures for management, as there is no solid scientific evidence that supports a benefit in visual outcomes.[33] Such measures include use of corticosteroids, cycloplegics, bilateral versus unilateral ocular patching, and bed rest versus light ambulation. Despite the limited evidence, recommended practice of supportive care includes elevation of the head of bed at least 30°, placement of a clear firm eye patch to prevent additional trauma, and restriction of physical activity. Although outpatient management can be cost effective, the ophthalmologist should decide between outpatient or inpatient management. This decision is based on concomitant injury, risk of rebleeding, IOP measurements, bleeding diathesis or sickle-cell disease, safety, likelihood of compliance, and access to medical care or follow-up.[31] Surgical management typically is undertaken if delayed complications emerge, rather than in the acute setting. However, patients with sickle-cell anemia or trait or with other specific concerns may undergo surgery sooner.[32] Otherwise, uncomplicated hyphemas tend to resolve within 4 or 5 days.[32]

Spontaneous hyphema should raise concern about underlying pathology, such as sickle-cell anemia, bleeding diatheses, herpes zoster, or ocular tumors.[12] In children with no predisposing disease or medication, the possibility of child abuse must be considered.[31]

RETINAL DETACHMENT

Retinal detachment (RD) is a relatively uncommon condition whereby the neurosensory retina separates and elevates from the retinal pigment epithelium (**Fig. 2**). When this occurs, the photoreceptor cells are separated from the choroidal blood supply,

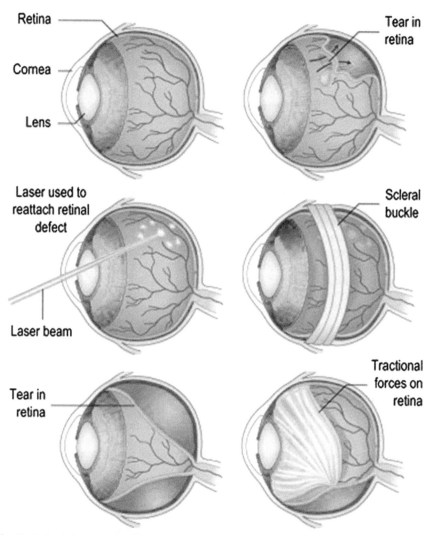

Fig. 2. Retinal detachment. (*From* Fisher SK, Lewis GP. Retinal detachment. In: Levin LA, Albert DM. Ocular disease: mechanisms and management. Philadelphia: Saunders; 2012. Chapter 71, p. 554–61; with permission.)

causing degeneration and anoxia and leading to loss of vision.[20] RD is classified into many types based on the underlying pathology. The incidence of RD is 10.1 per 100,000 per year, with 0.8% occurring secondary to trauma.[34] Penetrating injury to the globe carries a high risk of RD if the posterior segment is involved in a lacerating force, resulting in immediate retinal detachment. Blunt trauma can lead to RD by compression of the globe, with resultant tractional forces causing tears of the retina and subsequent separation of the vitreous gel.[2] In the setting of blunt trauma RD can occur acutely, but it typically occurs weeks to months after injury, with up to one-third of cases being diagnosed after 6 weeks.[13,35] This delay in development has been suggested to occur because solid vitreous gel internally tamponades the retina, so that breaks occurring acutely are stabilized. Over time, the vitreous may liquefy and dissect under the undetected retinal tear, causing the retina to detach.[10] Without a history of trauma, the most common form of RD is rhegmatogenous detachment, which results from predisposing degeneration of the retina, causing tears that detach via vitreoretinal traction.[2] Risk factors for the development of rhegmatogenous retinal detachment (RRD) include near-sightedness, family history (siblings are 3 times more likely to experience an RRD), and previous diagnosis of retinal detachment. In 15% of people with RD in one eye, it subsequently develops in the other eye.[20]

Symptoms of retinal detachment include unilateral floaters, photopsia (flashing light), and visual-field loss classically described as a "curtain" or "shadow" moving over the visual field.[3] The combination of new-onset floaters and flashing lights should be considered RD until proved otherwise. Typically this is a painless condition, and should be differentiated from symptoms that occur with migraines, which are usually bilateral flashes with associated headache.

Regardless of the precipitating events, examination of the eye should include assessment of visual acuity, visual fields, and pupillary response (afferent pupillary defect may be seen with retinal damage); ophthalmoscopy; and measurement of IOP (in the absence of suspected open-globe injury). Fundoscopic examination may reveal retinal breaks or vitreous hemorrhage. Imaging with ocular ultrasonography can detect a detached retina, which appears as a thick folded membrane that inserts into the optic disc.[36] In a small prospective observational study, Blaivas[29] found that emergency medicine physicians are able to accurately identify RD with bedside ultrasonography.

Management of RD in the ED is aimed at prompt recognition of the condition based on history and symptoms, and emergent referral to a retinal specialist. The prognosis depends on the involvement of the macula, size of the retinal tear, and duration of detachment.[12] An investigation that compared the prognosis of RD in adults secondary to open and closed ocular injury showed comparable outcomes, indicating that initial visual acuity and involvement of macula are the most prognostic indicators.[37] Surgery is the only treatment for established retinal detachment; therefore, prompt referral to an ophthalmologist is the most important aspect of ED management.

ACUTE-ANGLE CLOSURE GLAUCOMA

Various types of glaucoma have been described, each classified by underlying pathology and anatomy. Acute-angle closure glaucoma (AACG) is a vision-threatening condition whereby IOP increases, owing to blockage of aqueous circulation from the posterior chamber (where it is produced by the ciliary body) to the anterior chamber of the eye (where it is absorbed through the trabecular meshwork located within the angle).[10,16] When a cause is not found, the glaucoma is called primary angle closure glaucoma (PACG), which is most commonly caused by pupillary block.[38] In angle closure caused by pupillary block, the pupillary portion of the iris leaflet comes into contact with the lens, blocking aqueous flow from the posterior chamber of the eye through the pupil to the anterior chamber. The continuous production of aqueous humor is trapped within the posterior chamber, which pushes the iris anteriorly, further inhibiting outflow by narrowing the angle of the anterior chamber and obstructing the trabecular meshwork. This mechanism leads to acute increased IOP, which compromises vision by damaging the optic nerve or limiting vascular flow.[10]

AACG occurs in patients with anatomic predisposition, typically without a history of glaucoma, with narrow anterior-chamber angles.[2,16] Because of inherited predisposing features, the family history (especially among first-degree relatives) is a risk factor for development of the condition. Additional risk factors include increased age (due to increased lens size with aging), female gender, Asian race, and far-sightedness.[2,3,38] The condition can be precipitated by mydriasis, which occurs with accommodation, systemic anticholinergics, antipsychotics, or dim lighting.[3] The patient with AACG typically presents with acute-onset headache or monocular pain associated with blurred or cloudy vision, nausea, and vomiting. These symptoms can be misleading, and may be mistaken for abdominal abnormality or other causes of severe headache. It is therefore prudent to obtain a full history and to complete a thorough physical examination. The patient may also complain of classic "colored halos around lights," which are caused by corneal edema from increased IOP. Of importance, however, is that symptoms can be variable. Some patients have little pain despite high IOP, with the only symptom being decreased vision.[2] Physical examination findings of the affected eye classically include ciliary conjunctival injection, mid-dilated irregular and nonreactive pupil, and "steamy" cornea (due to edema).[12]

When AACG is suspected, the ocular examination should consist of visual acuity, pupil reactivity with pen light, slit-lamp examination, ophthalmoscopy, and measurement of IOP. In patients with AACG the pressure is remarkably elevated, typically greater than 21 mm Hg, and can range from 50 to 100 mm Hg.[12]

The goals of treatment are to reduce IOP and preserve visual function.[12] Definitive treatment requires rapid emergent referral to an ophthalmologist. Permanent visual loss may occur within hours, so ED management aimed at reducing IOP can be initiated while specialty consultation is being arranged.[3] The patient should be positioned supine to posteriorly shift the lens, which can assist in relieving pupillary block.[2] Production of aqueous humor can be reduced by topical agents, including β-blockers (eg, timolol 0.5%), α-agonists (eg, apraclonidine 1% or brimonidine 0.1%–0.2%), and/or steroids (eg, prednisolone acetate 1%). In addition, as long as the patient does not have contraindications, carbonic anhydrase inhibitors (such as acetazolamide) should be given. Nausea and pain should be managed with systemic antiemetics and analgesia. Hyperosmotic fluid, such as mannitol, is useful for quickly lowering IOP, and should be considered if other modalities are unsuccessful or if visual acuity is limited to detection of hand movements or worse.[3] Once IOP is reduced, a weak miotic, pilocarpine, 1% or 2%, should be applied to constrict the pupil and pull the iris away from the angle.[12] Definitive therapy provided by an ophthalmologist can include laser iridectomy or surgery. Because of anatomic predisposition, an untreated fellow eye has a 40% to 80% chance of developing AACG in 5 to 10 years. Typically ophthalmologists will treat the unaffected eye as well.[3,10]

SUMMARY

Any patient who presents to the ED with an ocular complaint requires a detailed history that includes the timing and onset of symptoms, and specific information regarding any trauma. In the setting of suspected trauma, a full and thorough examination must be performed to evaluate for possible intraocular foreign body, globe rupture, and hyphema, as these injuries are associated with complications and associated injuries. Most ocular injuries require definitive management by an ophthalmologist, but emergency physicians must be aware of temporizing measures that can reduce the risk of vision loss. Further studies are needed to provide evidence for clinical practice in the ED, so consultation with an ophthalmologist is always recommended in the setting of emergent ocular injuries and diseases.

ACKNOWLEDGMENTS

This article was copyedited by Linda J. Kesselring, MS, ELS, the technical editor/ writer in the Department of Emergency Medicine at the University of Maryland School of Medicine.

REFERENCES

1. Perry M, Dancey A, Mireskandari K, et al. Emergency care in facial trauma— a maxillofacial and ophthalmic perspective. Injury 2005;36(8):875–96.
2. Kanski JJ. Clinical ophthalmology. 6th edition. Edinburgh (United Kingdom): Elsevier Butterworth-Heinemann; 2007.
3. Ehlers JP, Shah CP. The Wills eye manual: office and emergency room diagnosis and treatment of eye disease. 5th edition. Philadelphia: Lippincott Williams & Wilkins; 2008.
4. Arey ML, Mootha VV, Whittemore AR, et al. Computed tomography in the diagnosis of occult open-globe injuries. Ophthalmology 2007;114(8):1448–52.
5. Hatton MP, Thakker MM, Ray S. Orbital and adnexal trauma associated with open-globe injuries. Ophthal Plast Reconstr Surg 2002;18(6):458–61.
6. Zhang Y, Zhang MN, Jiang CH, et al. Endophthalmitis following open globe injury. Br J Ophthalmol 2010;94(1):111–4.
7. Al-Mezaine HS, Osman EA, Kangave D, et al. Prognostic factors after repair of open globe injuries. J Trauma 2010;69(4):943–7.
8. Arnaiz J, Marco de Lucas E, Piedra T, et al. Intralenticular intraocular foreign body after stone impact: CT and US findings. Emerg Radiol 2006;12(5):237–9.
9. Raja SC, Goldberg MF. Injuries of the anterior segment. In: MacCumber M, editor. Management of ocular injuries and emergencies. Philadelphia: Lippincott-Raven; 1998. p. 227–34.
10. Fekrat S, MacCumber MW, Juan ED. Acute management of posterior segment injuries and emergencies. In: MacCumber M, editor. Management of ocular injuries and emergencies. Philadelphia: Lippincott-Raven; 1998. p. 285–307.
11. Yeh S, Colyer MH, Weichel ED. Current trends in the management of intraocular foreign bodies. Curr Opin Ophthalmol 2008;19(3):225–33.
12. Yanoff M. Ophthalmic clinical advisor: diagnosis and treatment. 2nd edition. St Louis (MO): Butterworth-Heinemann; 2008.
13. Bord SP, Linden J. Trauma to the globe and orbit. Emerg Med Clin North Am 2008;26(1):97–123.
14. Luo Z, Gardiner M. The incidence of intraocular foreign bodies and other intraocular findings in patients with corneal metal foreign bodies. Ophthalmology 2010; 117(11):2218–21.
15. Peate WF. Work-related eye injuries and illnesses. Am Fam Physician 2007;75(7): 1017–22.
16. Mitchell JD. Ocular emergencies. In: Tintinalli JE, Kelen GD, Stapczynski JS, editors. Emergency medicine: a comprehensive study guide. 6th edition. Upper Saddle River (NJ): Pearson/Prentice Hall; 2004. p. 1449.
17. Saeed A, Cassidy L, Malone DE, et al. Plain X-ray and computed tomography of the orbit in cases and suspected cases of intraocular foreign body. Eye 2008; 22(11):1373–7.
18. Adesanya OO, Dawkins DM. Intraorbital wooden foreign body (IOFB): mimicking air on CT. Emerg Radiol 2007;14(1):45–9.
19. Fulcher TP, McNab AA, Sullivan TJ. Clinical features and management of intraorbital foreign bodies. Ophthalmology 2002;109(3):494–500.

20. Chern K. Emergency ophthalmology: a rapid treatment guide. New York: McGraw-Hill, Medical Publishing Division; 2002.
21. Bhagat N, Nagori S, Zarbin M. Post-traumatic infectious endophthalmitis. Surv Ophthalmol 2011;56(3):214–51.
22. Vassallo S, Hartstein M, Howard D, et al. Traumatic retrobulbar hemorrhage: emergent decompression by lateral canthotomy and cantholysis. J Emerg Med 2002;22(3):251–6.
23. McClenaghan FC, Ezra DG, Holmes SB. Mechanisms and management of vision loss following orbital and facial trauma. Curr Opin Ophthalmol 2011;22(5): 426–31.
24. Shek KC, Chung KL, Kam CW, et al. Acute retrobulbar haemorrhage: an ophthalmic emergency. Emerg Med Australas 2006;18(3):299–301.
25. Popat H, Doyle PT, Davies SJ. Blindness following retrobulbar haemorrhage—it can be prevented. Br J Oral Maxillofac Surg 2007;45(2):163–4.
26. Winterton JV, Patel K, Mizen KD. Review of management options for a retrobulbar hemorrhage. J Oral Maxillofac Surg 2007;65(2):296–9.
27. Ghufoor K, Sandhu G, Sutcliffe J. Delayed onset of retrobulbar haemorrhage following severe head injury: a case report and review. Injury 1998;29(2):139–41.
28. Lima V, Burt B, Leibovitch I, et al. Orbital compartment syndrome: the ophthalmic surgical emergency. Surv Ophthalmol 2009;54(4):441–9.
29. Blaivas M. Bedside emergency department ultrasonography in the evaluation of ocular pathology. Acad Emerg Med 2000;7(8):947–50.
30. Sullivan TJ, Wright JE. Non-traumatic orbital haemorrhage. Clin Experiment Ophthalmol 2000;28(1):26–31.
31. Walton W, Von Hagen S, Grigorian R, et al. Management of traumatic hyphema. Surv Ophthalmol 2002;47(4):297–334.
32. Brandt MT, Haug RH. Traumatic hyphema: a comprehensive review. J Oral Maxillofac Surg 2001;59(12):1462–70.
33. Gharaibeh A, Savage HI, Scherer RW, et al. Medical interventions for traumatic hyphema. Cochrane Database Syst Rev 2011;(1):CD005431.
34. Sarrazin L, Averbukh E, Halpert M, et al. Traumatic pediatric retinal detachment: a comparison between open and closed globe injuries. Am J Ophthalmol 2004; 137(6):1042–9.
35. Pieramici DJ. Vitreoretinal trauma. Ophthalmol Clin North Am 2002;15(2):225–34.
36. Yoonessi R, Hussain A, Jang TB. Bedside ocular ultrasound for the detection of retinal detachment in the emergency department. Acad Emerg Med 2010;17(9): 913–7.
37. Rouberol F, Denis P, Romanet JP, et al. Comparative study of 50 early- or late-onset retinal detachments after open or closed globe injury. Retina 2011;31(6): 1143–9.
38. Pan Y, Varma R. Natural history of glaucoma. Indian J Ophthalmol 2011; 59(Suppl):S19–23.

Earache

Keith Conover, MD*

KEYWORDS

- Earache • Otitis • Mastoiditis • Tympanic membrane rupture • Cerumen impaction
- Foreign body

KEY POINTS

- A great variety of conditions, including some distant from the ear itself, may cause earache.
- Acute otitis media is diagnosed by a combination of signs and symptoms of acute otitis media (eg, fever, earache); and evidence of a middle ear effusion (fluid seen behind tympanic membrane, decreased mobility with insufflation by pneumatic otoscopy, opacity or discoloration of tympanic membrane not because of scarring, or evidence from tympanometry or spectral gradient acoustic reflectometry) but not simple redness of the tympanic membrane.
- Treating acute otitis media with antibiotics is controversial, with greatly varying yet prestigious guidelines of which patients to treat.
- Despite resistant organisms, high-dose amoxicillin, because of high concentrations in the middle ear, is still the drug of choice for acute otitis media.
- Malignant otitis externa is suspected in immunosuppressed patients with external ear erosions with visible bone, pain out of proportion to the physical examination, or an elevated erythrocyte sedimentation rate or an elevated white blood cell count, and may be confirmed by MRI.
- Perichondritis (infection of the external ear cartilage) is increasingly common because of upper ear piercing, may require incision and drainage, and requires systemic antibiotics covering *Pseudomonas* and methicillin-resistant *Staphylococcus aureus*.
- Ear candles should never be used.

OBJECTIVES

This article is designed to assist emergency physicians and other emergency department providers understand the following:

- The wide variety of conditions that may cause earache
- The principles of diagnosis of acute otitis media (AOM) and otitis media with effusion (OME)

Funding Sources: None.
Conflicts: None.
Department of Emergency Medicine, University of Pittsburgh, Suite 10028, Forbes Tower, PA 15260, USA
* 55 Sigrid Drive, Carnegie, PA 15106-3062.
E-mail address: kconover@pitt.edu

Emerg Med Clin N Am 31 (2013) 413–442
http://dx.doi.org/10.1016/j.emc.2013.02.001 **emed.theclinics.com**

- Emergency department treatment of AOM and OME
- Emergency department treatment of those with AOM and OME complicated by tympanostomy tubes or a ruptured tympanic membrane
- Recognition of the otitis media complications of mastoiditis and petrositis
- Treatment of acute traumatic tympanic membrane rupture
- Emergency department treatment of otitis externa and related conditions, including malignant otitis externa and cholesteatoma
- The increasing incidence and treatment of perichondritis
- Appropriate treatment of cerumen impaction, with attention to those with diabetes mellitus or other immunocompromise and anticoagulation
- Issues in the removal of foreign bodies from the external ear

EARACHE

Earache is very common. For example, 80% of children in Boston have otitis media before age 3 years.[1] In 1990, there were 25 million medical visits for AOM.[2] In 1986, the indirect cost of otitis media was estimated at $3.5 billion.[3]

An immunization for *Haemophilus influenzae* type B has been used throughout the developed world since about 1980; however, most of the *H influenzae* found in AOM cannot be typed, meaning that the *H influenzae* type B vaccine has not affected the incidence of AOM. However, pediatric visits to primary care offices, urgent care centers, and emergency departments for otitis media decreased by a third after the introduction and widespread use of a pneumonia (*Streptococcus pneumoniae* [pneumococcus]) vaccine in 2000.[4,5] Still, that leaves a lot of visits, and this does not count otitis externa or all the other causes of earache. In one study, two-thirds of earache was caused by ear problems, such as AOM or otitis externa, but one-third were referred pain, and given the complex innervation of the ear this pain was referred from a variety of sources.[6]

Some of the more common causes for earache other than otitis media, otitis externa, or barotrauma (incidence >100/100,000)[7] in order of frequency include the following.[8,9] Additional lists of even less common causes of ear pain may be found in the literature.[9]

- Carious or abscessed teeth
- Temporomandibular joint (TMJ) pain, either from an acute posttraumatic TMJ capsulitis (contusion of the cartilage of the jaw joint) or chronic TMJ pain
- Cervical spine pain
- Cervical lymphadenitis (swollen infected lymph nodes in the neck)
- Tonsillitis
- Posttonsillectomy pain
- Acute parotitis (inflammation of the parotid salivary gland in the cheek from viral, bacterial, or noninfectious causes)

Assume one looks at the outside of the ear, and then looks at the inside of the ear with an otoscope, and everything looks normal. The earache is worse with range of motion of the jaw, or with biting down. There is tenderness just anterior to the tragus of the ear, where one can feel the TMJ, especially with range of motion of the jaw. If after a blow to the jaw, even on the other side, it is likely acute posttraumatic TMJ capsulitis, or perhaps a tear of the cartilage meniscus in the TMJ; if more chronic, it may be TMJ syndrome.

If the ear looks normal, but on oral examination there is tap tenderness of a nearby tooth, especially if there is visual evidence of caries or abscess, then that is likely the cause of the earache. Earache with a normal ear examination but tender cervical lymph nodes below the ear indicates cervical lymphadenitis, which may cause pain interpreted as earache.

It is very common for people to have sore throat and earache. If the ear examination is normal, it is likely tonsillar pain radiating to the ears. Sometimes people present primarily with an earache, but a normal ear examination and with only minor throat pain, but with tonsillitis on oral examination. Even a lingual tonsillitis, hard or impossible to see on examination of the oropharynx, may cause pain referred to the ear. Peritonsillar cellulitis or abscess may cause severe unilateral ear pain with a normal ear examination.

Posttonsillectomy pain commonly radiates to the ears. Serous middle ear effusions are common after tonsillectomy. Ear pain with a normal examination, but with swelling and pain in the distribution of the parotid salivary gland, suggests parotitis. Parotitis may be a viral or bacterial infection or noninfectious, including such problems as an obstructive stone in Stensen duct.

OTITIS MEDIA
AOM (Acute Suppurative Otitis Media)

AOM is distinguished from other forms of otitis media, including OME (otitis media with effusion, secretory otitis media, serous otitis, "glue ear") and chronic otitis media (chronic suppurative otitis media). Chronic otitis media is now rare in developed countries, thanks to the introduction of antibiotics in the 1930s. Some also define other types of otitis media, such as persistent and recurrent AOM and recurrent OME.[10] AOM often occurs coincident with, or subsequent to, an episode of acute viral rhinosinusitis (a cold).[11] Although now generally regarded as a relatively benign condition, in the era before antibiotics sequelae and complications were common.[10]

Diagnosis of AOM

AOM is defined as the presence of fluid in the middle ear in association with signs or symptoms of acute local or systemic illness. Accompanying signs and symptoms may be specific for AOM, such as otalgia or otorrhea; or nonspecific, such as fever.[12] With this general statement, the diagnosis of AOM is clearly defined and agreed on, but the specific diagnostic criteria remain elusive. One survey of 165 pediatricians resulted in 147 different sets of criteria, and in 26 clinical trials 18 different sets of criteria were used.[13]

Diagnosing a middle ear effusion is relatively straightforward. Pneumatic otoscopy is recommended, looking for position, color, translucency, and mobility.[12] In one study, as confirmed by myringotomy, pneumatic otoscopy was 93% sensitive and 58% specific, which compares favorably with tympanometry, which was 90% sensitive and 86% specific.[14]

A 2004 clinical guideline on OME states: "Distinct redness of the tympanic membrane should not be a criterion for antibiotic prescribing because it has poor predictive value for AOM and is present in about 5% of ears with OME."[15] A red tympanic membrane may also be a result of crying or irritation from removing cerumen.[16] A retracted tympanic membrane, which may be painful, is caused by negative middle ear pressure, likely the result of eustachian tube dysfunction and not of a bacterial infection.[11]

One recent study used the following definition of middle ear effusion: two or more of decreased or absent tympanic membrane mobility, yellow or white discoloration of the tympanic membrane, opacification of the tympanic membrane not caused by scarring, and visible bubbles or air-fluid levels.[17]

Pelton[18] tabulates a multivariate analysis of how three findings (color, position, and mobility) correlate with AOM determined by myringotomy. The combination of a cloudy tympanic membrane, a bulging tympanic membrane, and a tympanic membrane with slightly or distinctly impaired mobility correlated highly with AOM (99%). The full predictive values and associated findings are reproduced in **Table 1**, sorted by predictive value. Note that pneumatic otoscopy to determine mobility adds significantly to the predictive value of the examination.

The development of machines that assess for middle ear effusion without a prolonged fight with a squirming, screaming infant to perform pneumatic otoscopy, or worse, digging wax out of the ear of a squirming, screaming infant before performing pneumatic otoscopy, seemed to be attractive to many physicians. Tympanometry uses a mechanical device to measure features of the tympanic membrane and middle ear, and can assess for middle ear effusion. Tympanometry has been available since the early 1970s. Tympanometers are simple to use, although results are a bit complex to interpret. They are found in many otolaryngology offices and some pediatric offices and emergency departments.

First-generation tympanometers assess the tympanic membrane and middle ear by measuring the quantity of a 226-Hz musical tone reflected back from the tympanic membrane as a function of how the air pressure in the external canal is varied above and below ambient air pressure. Second-generation tympanometers use a pair of musical tones. The tympanometer plots a pressure-versus-compliance curve on a graph known as a tympanogram. Different curves strongly suggest certain anatomic correlates in the middle ear, such as tympanic membrane thinning (eg, healed postrupture) or ossicular disarticulation; middle ear effusion versus ossicular fixation; middle ear effusion; sclerosis; cerumen impaction; or retracted tympanic membrane. The interpretation of tympanograms is described in the medical literature and in other sources but is beyond the scope of this article.[19,20] There is no evidence

Table 1
Predictive values of physical examination findings for acute otitis media

Predictive Value (%)	Color	Position	Mobility
99	Cloudy	Bulging	Distinctly impaired
99	Cloudy	Bulging	Slightly impaired
97	Cloudy	Normal	Distinctly impaired
94	Distinctly red	Bulging	Distinctly impaired
94	Cloudy	Normal	Distinctly impaired
93	Slightly red	Bulging	Slightly impaired
89	Distinctly red	Normal	Distinctly impaired
85	Slightly red	Bulging	Distinctly impaired
83	Distinctly red	Bulging	Slightly impaired
47	Distinctly red	Normal	Slightly impaired
41	Slightly red	Normal	Slightly impaired
37	Cloudy	Normal	Normal
29	Normal	Retracted	Distinctly impaired
15	Distinctly red	Normal	Normal
7	Slightly red	Normal	Normal
3	Normal	Retracted	Slightly impaired
0.1	Normal	Normal	Normal

that tympanometry is superior to pneumatic otoscopy for diagnosing middle ear effusion.

Tympanometry requires an airtight seal between the instrument and the external ear canal; however, a newer related technique, spectral gradient acoustic reflectometry (SGAR), does not require such a seal. SGAR machines emit a series of tones in a spectrum from 1.8 to 4.4 kHz, and measure the reflectance of the different frequency tones. The patterns may be mapped to curves known to be characteristic of certain middle ear conditions, including middle ear effusion. As with tympanometry, accuracy is dependent on user technique.[21]

A 1999 article provides a detailed and critical review of studies of tympanometry and SGAR up to that point, and concluded that although tympanometry and SGAR might be useful tools in certain settings, they do not supplant history, physical examination, and pneumatic otoscopy for the diagnosis of AOM.[22] A 2007 study found SGAR almost as good as tympanometry at distinguishing middle ear effusion, and pointed out the advantages of SGAR over tympanometry: "unlike tympanometry, SGAR can be performed in relatively uncooperative children and its successful performance does not depend, as does that of tympanometry, on achieving an airtight seal between the instrument and the walls of the external auditory canal."[17] Acoustic reflectometry can distinguish a middle ear effusion, but cannot distinguish OME from AOM.[23] The accuracy of reflectometry depends on the design of the reflectometer, with more recent designs being superior to older ones.[24]

Thus, despite problems dealing with cerumen in the canal obscuring the tympanic membrane, and uncooperative infants, pneumatic otoscopy is still slightly superior to tympanometry and SGAR for diagnosing middle ear effusion, one of the requirements for diagnosing AOM. As Combs[25] writes: "No technology can replace the careful history and otoscopic examination by an experienced physician."

Parents often present with a child and concerns about AOM. Although physicians are unable to diagnosis AOM by symptoms alone, parents are able to do so with a sensitivity of 71% and specificity of 80%.[26]

Antibiotics for AOM?

In the 1980s, it was said that "any child with an earache has an acute amoxicillin deficiency until proven otherwise." Tradition is powerful, and the tradition in the United States (and Australia) is that if parents bring in a child with an earache, the clinician will prescribe antibiotics. However, in parts of Europe, AOM is not treated with antibiotics as often.[27,28] In the Netherlands, antibiotics are prescribed for 31% to 56% of children with AOM[29,30]; in the United States the rate is 95%.[31]

It used to be taught that antibiotics were appropriate, at least in younger children, to decrease the incidence of deafness, known to be caused by otitis media. However, permanent deafness comes primarily from chronic suppurative otitis media (2 or more weeks of otitis media with discharge), which is quite rare in developed countries. AOM does not cause such deafness, although lingering effusions may cause temporary partial deafness.[32] More serious complications of otitis media, such as permanent deafness or death from brain infection by contiguous spread, are also primarily a problem of the developing world, particularly of eastern Asia and the western Pacific, where it represents a significant medical burden.[33] However, chronic suppurative otitis media and its complications are quite rare in developed countries.[34] The reason for this difference is unclear.[33]

In the developed world, the past four decades has seen the traditional antibiotic treatment of AOM increasingly called into question. There are concerns about creating resistant bacteria, and questions about the efficacy of antibiotics for AOM.[35]

In recent years in the United States has it been acceptable to delay treating pediatric AOM with antibiotics, at least for some patients, opting to treat with analgesics instead (delayed antibiotics or observation). The clinician provides a prescription for an antibiotic (a safety-net antibiotic prescription[36]), but also gives instructions to not fill it unless the pain continues for more than a day or so. Frequently, the earache ceases, and then there is no perceived need to fill the prescription. This has been shown to provide parent satisfaction and decrease the number of prescriptions filled,[36,37] which it is hoped will delay the emergence of resistant bacteria, not to mention preventing adverse effects from the antibiotics. Some parents are convinced that their child needs antibiotics and fill the prescription right away. However, in most pediatric studies satisfaction is the same whether the parents are given a prescription or told to call back or return if their child is not better in 2 to 3 days, and fewer children get antibiotics if the patient is discharged without a prescription.[38,39] A large 2001 study found that an immediate antibiotic reduces crying during the day and sleep disturbances at night the first day, and decreases acetaminophen use. This occurs after the first day, when symptoms are already diminishing. However, some argue that such a minimal benefit may not outweigh adverse effects of the antibiotic nor the risk of creating resistant bacterial strains.[40] For adult patients with AOM, delayed prescribing has not been studied.

The medical literature is filled with articles debating the merits of antibiotics for children with otitis media in general, and the subset of those who should receive antibiotics, and in particular, whether antibiotics are indicated for those younger than 2 years of age.[35,41–48] However, a recent (March 2008) international conference of experts was unable to achieve a consensus on when antibiotics are appropriate for otitis media.[49]

There are presently two competing prestigious recommendations for how to treat AOM. The American Academy of Pediatrics (AAP) and the American Academy of Family Physicians (AAFP) released a joint clinical practice guideline on the management of AOM in 2004.[50] It has had limited impact on prescribing practices.[51,52] The primary recommendations of this guideline are as follows:

- To diagnose AOM the clinician should confirm a history of acute onset, identify signs of middle ear effusion, and evaluate for the presence of signs and symptoms of middle ear inflammation.
- The management of AOM should include an assessment of pain. If pain is present, the clinician should recommend treatment to reduce pain.
- Observation without use of antibacterial agents in a child with uncomplicated AOM is an option for selected children based on diagnostic certainty, age, illness severity, and assurance of follow-up. (The guideline recommends that those younger than 6 months of age, with a certain or uncertain diagnosis of AOM, be treated with antibiotics immediately; from 6 months to 2 years of age, that immediate antibiotics be started if the diagnosis is certain, or if the diagnosis is uncertain and there is severe illness; and that for those older than 2 years age, observation is an option, whether diagnosis is certain or uncertain, as long as there is no severe illness.)
- If a decision is made to treat with an antibacterial agent, the clinician should prescribe amoxicillin for most children. When amoxicillin is used, the dose should be 80 to 90 mg/kg/d (high dose). In patients who have severe illness (moderate to severe otalgia or fever of $\geq 39°C$) and in those for whom additional coverage for β-lactamase–positive *H influenzae* and *Moraxella catarrhalis* is desired, therapy should be initiated with high-dose amoxicillin-clavulanate (90 mg/kg/d of

amoxicillin component, with 6.4 mg/kg/d of clavulanate in two divided doses). If the patient is allergic to amoxicillin and the allergic reaction was not a type I hypersensitivity reaction (urticaria or anaphylaxis), cefdinir (14 mg/kg/d in one or two doses), cefpodoxime (10 mg/kg/d, once daily), or cefuroxime (30 mg/kg/d in two divided doses) can be used. In cases of type I reactions, azithromycin (10 mg/kg/d on Day 1 followed by 5 mg/kg/d for 4 days as a single daily dose) or clarithromycin (15 mg/kg/d in two divided doses) can be used to select an antibacterial agent of an entirely different class. Other possibilities include erythromycin-sulfisoxazole (50 mg/kg/d of erythromycin) or sulfamethoxazole-trimethoprim (6–10 mg/kg/d of trimethoprim). Alternative therapy in the penicillin-allergic patient who is being treated for infection that is known or presumed to be caused by penicillin-resistant S pneumoniae is clindamycin at 30 to 40 mg/kg/d in three divided doses. In the patient who is vomiting or cannot otherwise tolerate oral medication, a single dose of parenteral ceftriaxone (50 mg/kg) has been shown to be effective for the initial treatment of AOM.
- If the patient fails to respond to the initial management option within 48 to 72 hours, the clinician must reassess the patient to confirm AOM and exclude other causes of illness. If AOM is confirmed in the patient initially managed with observation, the clinician should begin antibacterial therapy. If the patient was initially managed with an antibacterial agent, the clinician should change the antibacterial agent.

The respected Cochrane Review of antibiotics for AOM in children,[53] however, representing a more cosmopolitan perspective than the United States-only AAP-AAFP guideline, was updated in 2010. It notes that antibiotics slightly decrease pain at 24 hours and for a few days following, and that delayed antibiotic prescribing worked as well as immediate antibiotics. It notes that antibiotics made no difference in recurrence or more severe complications, such as temporary deafness, rupture of the tympanic membrane, or mastoiditis. However, complications from the antibiotic (vomiting, diarrhea, and rash) were common (37%). The Cochrane Review concludes that antibiotics should not be used for most cases of AOM, and are appropriate only if there is bilateral AOM or there is AOM with otorrhea (discharge from the ear).

The Cochrane review and the AAP-AAFP guidelines are based on essentially the same evidence, which is primarily from developed countries. They do take into account different traditions and public expectations, and interpret the balance of risks and benefits differently. In essence, both recommend only treating severe AOM with antibiotics; the 2010 Cochrane review considers severe to be restricted to bilateral AOM or AOM with otorrhea, whereas the 2004 AAP-AAFP guideline takes a much more inclusive view of what is severe, including any patient younger than age 2, or especially younger than 6 months of age. It is hard to see how one could be accused of practicing bad medicine if one follows either of these two prestigious guidelines.

Even though many bacteria isolated from ears with AOM are resistant to amoxicillin, amoxicillin is still recommended as first-line treatment because it is as clinically effective as other antibiotics.[38,39] A single dose of intramuscular ceftriaxone and 5 days of oral azithromycin are as effective as amoxicillin.[54] There has been an increasing incidence of multidrug-resistant S pneumoniae (pneumococcus) in AOM. There are many recommendations, therefore, to switch from standard-dose amoxicillin (25–50 mg/kg/d divided twice a day or three times a day, maximum 30 mg/kg/day if child is <3 months old) to high-dose amoxicillin (80–90 mg/kg/d divided twice a day). This achieves high concentrations in the middle ear, which is not the case for oral cephalosporins, which is one reason that amoxicillin is still recommended as first-line treatment of AOM. The AAP-AAFP guideline summarized previously provides guidance for cases of penicillin allergy. Although twice-a-day dosing is often used, a Cochrane Review concluded that there is not enough evidence to support twice-a-day dosing instead of three times a day.[55] Courses of antibiotics shorter than 7 days have been reviewed by the Cochrane Collaboration, and because of a higher failure rate, are not recommended.[56]

Resistant AOM (persistence of fever, otalgia, and red, bulging tympanic membranes or persistent otorrhea after 3 or more days of antibiotic therapy) should be treated with high-dose amoxicillin–clavulanate, cefuroxime axetil, or intramuscular ceftriaxone for 3 days, according to one expert panel.[57] No evidence-based recommendations for resistant AOM are yet available. Patients with resistant AOM should be encouraged to follow-up with a primary care physician as soon as possible.

Recurrent AOM (a repeat episode occurring a month after the initial episode) is almost always (>90%) from a new pathogen.[58] There are some recommendations in the literature to suggest that amoxicillin-clavulanate is the appropriate first choice for such episodes. Having an episode of AOM before age 6 months is associated with recurrent episodes of AOM. However, there seems to be no association with day care, gender, familial history of allergy, duration of breast-feeding, or domestic environment.[59] Recurrent AOM tends to resolve as children grow older.[60] There is some evidence that prophylactic antibiotics, either throughout the cold season or with onset of a viral upper respiratory infection, may help prevent AOM in children with a history of recurrent episodes.[61]

One final note about antibiotics. When a parent or guardian says "amoxicillin never works for his/her ear infections!" I believe them. Some kids are probably colonized with amoxicillin-resistant bacteria. Scientific studies are not good enough yet to tease out these outliers. So, I prescribe something else, and call it the art of medicine.

Other Treatments for AOM

Oral decongestants and antihistamines have been studied for AOM, and based on multiple studies a Cochrane review recommends against them. There was slight benefit with a combination of oral decongestants and antihistamines, but the side effects outweigh the minimal benefit.[62] A recent study finds no benefits at all from antihistamines, decongestants, or both combined.[63] One older study found that a combination of antihistamine and decongestant taken during acute viral rhinosinusitis (a cold) did not prevent subsequent AOM.[64]

Interestingly, a recent study showed a trend toward benefit, not from oral decongestants or antihistamines, but from a topical decongestant (nasal spray): approximately 27% resolution of effusion at 1 month as opposed to 19% resolution for decongestants, antihistamines, or controls.[63] A short course of oxymetazoline (Afrin) nasal spray (<10 days to avoid rhinitis medicamentosa, which one can describe to patients as "being addicted to nasal spray so you have to use it to breathe through your nose") seems appropriate.[65,66] For otitis media or OME, I tell patients to spray into both nostrils, then lie flat on their backs for a few minutes, so that they can taste the spray getting back to where the eustachian tubes drain out in the back of the nose and throat.

One study showed a modest amount of pain control from an ear drop consisting of glycerin, antipyrine, and benzocaine (Auralgan).[67] A Cochrane review of various types of analgesic ear drops concluded that there was not enough evidence to know if they are effective.[68]

Otitis-Conjunctivitis Syndrome

Conjunctivitis and otitis media are sometimes found together, and the combination is highly likely to be caused by *H influenzae*.[69] *H influenzae* tends to be resistant to antibiotics commonly used for ear infections, such as amoxicillin and azithromycin (Zithromax); therefore, it is important to look for conjunctivitis that might indicate a need for a different antibiotic.[70–73] Amoxicillin-clavulanate (Augmentin), cefuroxime (Ceftin), and cefdinir (Omnicef) are commonly prescribed antibiotics that cover resistant H influenzae.[74]

If examining a patient with purulent conjunctivitis, it is worthwhile examining the ears; roughly two-thirds also have AOM, and thus should be prescribed an oral antibiotic rather than eyedrops.[75] If one is prescribing oral antibiotics, there is generally no need to prescribe antibiotic eye drops for uncomplicated conjunctivitis; the tears are thought to contain adequate amounts of the systemic antibiotics, lasting much longer than eyedrops between doses, and serve the same purpose adequately.[76]

Otitis Media with Effusion (Glue Ear, Serous Otitis, Middle Ear Effusion)

Sometimes in the emergency department one sees a patient with a complaint solely of decreased hearing. When one looks in the ear, rather than a cerumen impaction, one sees an ear that has a clear effusion, fluid behind the tympanic membrane. Or, one may routinely examine an ear and see some fluid behind the tympanic membrane.

It is common for a middle ear effusion to persist after AOM. At 2 weeks after AOM, about three-fourth of children have a persistent effusion; a month after, half do; and 3 months later, 10% to 25% do. This is not an indication for additional antibiotics.[1,12,77]

OME may also less commonly result from eustachian tube dysfunction from other causes, such chronic eustachian tube deformity, environmental allergies,[78] tobacco smoking, and esophageal reflux.[79] OME may cause discomfort, decreased hearing, or a feeling of "water in the ear." OME is defined as fluid in the middle ear without signs or symptoms of acute ear infection, and as with AOM, is primarily a problem of children.[15] OME may cause significantly decreased hearing, resulting in decreased scores in tests of speech and cognitive abilities, which is why it is a particular focus for pediatric primary care.[80]

In the emergency department, a cloudy TM, a visible effusion with an air-fluid level, or bubbles behind the tympanic membrane without symptoms of acute infection is also sufficient to tentatively establish the diagnosis and refer for outpatient follow-up. A 2004 clinical guideline of The AAP, AAFP, and American Academy of Otolaryngology–Head and Neck Surgery recommends pneumatic otoscopy to identify OME. Although optional in the emergency department, decreased mobility with insufflation confirms the diagnosis.[50]

Unfortunately, for patients in the emergency department with OME, there is little that can be done. Studies show that autoinflation with a Politzer device, antihistamines, decongestants, steroids, and antibiotics are all essentially useless.[15,81–84] One mucolytic proved worse than useless.[85] The AAP, AAFP, and American Academy of Otolaryngology–Head and Neck Surgery guideline recommends as initial management for children (2 months to 12 years of age) with OME a 3-month period of "watchful waiting," checking hearing tests, and considering tympanostomy tubes.[15]

OME, although primarily a disease of children, also occurs in adults. Causative factors of cases referred to otolaryngologists include chronic sinus disease (particularly of the ethmoids); tobacco smoking; adenoidal hyperplasia; sequelae of AOM; and rarely head and neck tumors (<5% of cases).[86] There is strong suspicion that many cases of OME are caused by allergy, but controlled treatment studies are lacking.[87] Emergency department management consists primarily of referral to an otolaryngologist. In cases where allergy seems a likely cause, it is reasonable to treat for this with a nonsedating antihistamine and a steroid nasal spray. For those with OME after AOM, or from acute viral rhinosinusitis, given the findings for AOM[63] a short course of oxymetazoline (Afrin) nasal spray (<10 days to avoid rhinitis medicamentosa) is appropriate.[65,66] Simple anatomic considerations lead to a recommendation for patients to lie supine for a few minutes after using a nasal spray for OME.

AOM with Tympanostomy Tube or Ruptured Tympanic Membrane

Tympanostomy tubes (myringotomy tubes, ventilation tubes, "grommets") are sometimes surgically inserted in the tympanic membranes of children with recurrent AOM or, particularly in children older than 3 years, chronic OME. It is common to have otorrhea for days to a few weeks after insertion of tympanostomy tubes, and this is considered a normal consequence of the surgical procedure.

There may be a question as to whether a patient who has had tympanostomy tubes in the past, or who has otorrhea and one cannot see the tympanic membrane, might have a perforation in the tympanic membrane. Any patient who can taste ear drops when administered, or who can expel air out their ear canal with pinched-nose blowing, should be assumed to have a perforation.[88]

About 5% of children with tubes develop chronic otorrhea (drainage from the ear), usually caused by skin flora, such as *Pseudomonas aeruginosa* and *Staphylococcus aureus*.[89] Infants and children with tympanostomy tubes not uncommonly present to the emergency department with acute otorrhea. This occurs in roughly half of children with tubes.[90] From the otorrhea, the external ear canal may acquire an eczematous appearance.[88] Usually there are minimal associated symptoms: low-grade temperature and fatigue, but seldom pain.

In one study, approximately 30% of children with AOM had a spontaneous rupture of the tympanic membrane during an episode of AOM; this was more common if they had a history of prior AOM. Almost always there is a sudden decrease in pain. Eighty-five percent of the ruptures were in the anteroinferior portion, with smooth margins, and provided adequate drainage. In the other 15% the rupture was in the posterosuperior portion of the TM, and was small and nipple-like. Ninety-four percent of the perforations were spontaneously healed within a month. Children who have had a perforation are twice as likely to have recurrent AOM.[91]

The bacteriology of intermittent otorrhea with tubes in those younger than age 3 is essentially the same as that for AOM in this group: a mixture of viruses and airway-derived bacteria.[92,93] In older children, it is usually skin flora including *P aeruginosa* and *S aureus*.[94]

There are a wide range of treatments of such otorrhea, from simple observation without treatment, to topical antibiotics (ear drops), to systemic antibiotics. In children younger than 3 years old with acute tube-associated otorrhea, one study found ear drops as effective as oral antibiotics; however, oral antibiotics were provided for those with fever or significant ear pain or failure of ear drops.[92] One study found ofloxacin ear drops (Floxin) as effective as oral amoxicillin-clavulanate.[95] Given that ear drops are effective for tube-associated otorrhea in all ages of infants and children, it seems prudent to use ear drops as the initial treatment for all such children, unless there is severe ear pain or high fever, in which case ear drops (to cover skin flora) and oral antibiotics should be prescribed.[96]

At times ear drops go through tympanostomy tubes into the middle ear, depending on a variety of factors. There is enough concern for ototoxicity that it is recommended that only nonototoxic eardrops be used when there are tympanostomy tubes or a possible tympanic membrane perforation.[97] Aminoglycoside antibiotics and propylene glycol have been found to be ototoxic in animal studies.[98,99] It is also recommended that ear drops with alcohol or with a low pH be avoided in such cases, because of concerns about pain and ototoxicity.[88] Chloramphenicol ear drops with propylene glycol are not readily available in the United States; however, they may be available from foreign countries, and if patients enquire about their use, it is best to recommend against them and prescribe an alternative. Neomycin and polymyxin B and hydrocortisone otic suspension (Cortisporin) contains an aminoglycoside (neomycin) and propylene glycol,[98] and acetic acid ear drops (Vosol, Acetasol; Vosol-HC, Acetasol-HC) also contain propylene glycol, so they should not be used for tube-associated otorrhea (or perforated tympanic membranes) unless the risks outweigh the benefits.

Ciprofloxacin-dexamethasone (Ciprodex) has been found to be nonototoxic in an animal model.[100] In company-supported research, it has been shown to result in some-what faster resolution of tube-associated otorrhea than ofloxacin ear drops (Floxin).[101] There is some independent evidence that adding a steroid to an antibiotic results in faster resolution of external otitis, and a steroid alone is effective even without an antibiotic.[102,103]

In the rare case of a child with tubes presenting to the emergency department with ongoing otorrhea refractory to appropriate ear drops, it is appropriate to obtain a culture, allowing the follow-up provider to use culture results to guide treatment, but not change treatment in the emergency department. If the patient is now having significant ear pain or fever, it is appropriate to start oral antibiotics after culturing.[92]

Mastoiditis and Petrositis

A hundred years ago, mastoiditis and petrositis were common and dreaded complications of otitis media: 20% of patients with otitis media got mastoiditis or petrositis. However, these complications became much less common (2%), and especially rare in the developed world (<1%), after antibiotics became available in the 1930s.[104] The incidence is somewhat higher in the Netherlands, where antibiotics are much less commonly prescribed for AOM.[28]

Mastoiditis is best described as symptomatic infection of the air cells in the bony mastoid process behind the ear. It is most common in those younger than 2 years old.[105] The classic presentation of mastoiditis, swelling and perhaps warmth or redness over the mastoid, with anterior and inferior displacement of the pinna, is now seldom seen. Antibiotics may obscure the usual symptoms of mastoiditis; there are reports of "masked mastoiditis" where patients develop further complications of mastoiditis, such as brain abscess, without classic signs of mastoiditis.[106] Masked mastoiditis reports date back to 1941, soon after initial use of antibiotics for otitis media.[107] The most common findings are now an abnormality of the tympanic membrane and sagging of the posterior wall of the external ear canal.[10] Beers and coworkers[108] also suggest looking behind the ear, because sometimes in mastoiditis the postauricular fold is obliterated; compare with the unaffected side.

The diagnostic criteria for mastoiditis are poorly defined.[109] As with fluid in the sinuses on computed tomography (CT) that occurs with most any viral upper respiratory infection,[110–112] fluid in the mastoid air cells on CT is nondiagnostic, found in many cases of otitis media.[113] High-resolution CT findings of bony resorption in the mastoid, combined with some clinical signs of mastoiditis, permits a diagnosis of "coalescent" mastoiditis, which is simply another way of saying the bony septae between the mastoid air cells are being destroyed.[114] Suspected cases of mastoiditis should be imaged (CT or magnetic resonance imaging [MRI]) because findings of "coalescent" mastoiditis may be diagnostic. However, there are no other accepted criteria for CT or MRI diagnosis of mastoiditis.[109] A visual review of the CT findings of mastoiditis and related conditions is available in print and online.[115]

Patients with mastoiditis are generally admitted for further work-up and treatment. Myringotomy is usually performed and tympanostomy tubes are generally placed. If there are neither subperiosteal abscess nor central nervous system involvement, a period of 48 hours of observation and broad-spectrum intravenous (IV) antibiotics is recommended before considering mastoidectomy.[116] Subperiosteal abscesses are surgically drained.

Petrositis (infection of the petrous portion of the temporal bone, Gradenigo syndrome) was classically described as presenting with the triad of deep facial pain, otitis media, and ipsilateral abducens nerve paralysis.[117] However, such classic presentations are rare today; a history of chronic otitis media or surgery for mastoiditis with ongoing symptoms of infection, and deep facial pain, which is the single unifying symptom in a series of eight modern cases, should increase one's suspicion for petrositis.[118]

Suspected cases of petrositis should be imaged (CT or MRI), and are generally admitted for further work-up and treatment. CT findings of bony changes in the petrous area are diagnostic.[118] Although mastoidectomy is a common treatment, there are case reports of successful conservative management of adults and children with just antibiotics.[119–121]

Facial Nerve Paralysis

Facial nerve paralysis is a rare complication of AOM in adults and in children. The causes are unclear. There are recommendations in the literature that this should be managed conservatively with antibiotics and steroids, and that the time course for the paralysis is generally 2 weeks to 3 months.[122–124]

Bullous Myringitis

Bullous myringitis used to be thought to indicate infection with mycoplasma.[125] More recently it has been found that, except for a slight increase in S pneumoniae, the pathogens in those with bullous myringitis are the same as for any case of AOM.[126] Bullous myringitis is associated with worse AOM and more severe pain.[126] As one review put it, bullous myringitis is just AOM with blisters on the eardrum.[125]

BAROTRAUMA AND TRAUMATIC TYMPANIC PERFORATION

Traumatic perforation of the tympanic membrane may occur secondary to a blow to the ear (the most common cause in one series,[127] mostly from domestic violence or street fights); blast injury (including fireworks); barotrauma from diving or altitude exposure; or direct trauma to the tympanic membrane. Symptoms of tympanic membrane perforations are generally fullness, tinnitus, or hearing loss. Any patient with severe vertigo after a ruptured tympanic membrane may have a perilymphatic fistula or rupture of the round window, and an otolaryngologist should be consulted urgently for such patients.[128] Approximately 90% of civilian perforations heal in a month with no specific treatment.[127,129] Explosion-related blast injuries from war tend to be larger; to be similarly symptomatic (83%); and not to heal spontaneously as frequently (48%).[130] There is evidence from the 1974 Birmingham bombings that very large perforations (80% or more of the TM) do not heal spontaneously, and that smaller perforations (<80%) tend to heal spontaneously; there is a recommendation to allow a month for healing of each 10% of the tympanic membrane that is lost.[131]

For at least 2 weeks after a perforation, it is strongly recommended that there be no cleaning or instrumentation of the external ear canal, unless there is visible contamination or evidence of infection, in which case it is recommended to use gentle suction and mopping to remove debris.[132] There is no evidence that ear drops improve healing of traumatic tympanic membrane perforations. There are opinions, based on large observational series where healing occurred at a high rate despite the lack of such ear drops, that they are not needed.[127] There are also expert opinions in the literature that ear drops are not helpful and may well be harmful.[132] There is some evidence, albeit with small numbers, that worse healing is associated with the use of ear drops (2 of 9 with ear drops healed at 4 weeks vs 29 of 33 healed at 4 weeks with no ear drops), and ear irrigation and antibiotic ear drops seem to be associated with increased infection rates.[132] Because moisture in the ear seems to make infection more likely, it is recommended that patients be carefully instructed to keep the ear dry. There are a few recommendations that an infected ruptured tympanic membrane be treated with oral antibiotics, but this is not evidence-based and there is neither evidence nor expert recommendations as to the appropriate antibiotics.[127] Given the experience with otorrhea with tympanostomy tubes (see later), coverage for *P aeruginosa* and methicillin-resistant *S aureus* (MRSA) is appropriate.

Advice from a Canadian otolaryngologist from World War II still seems to the point. *The correct treatment of recent rupture of a drum in the forward areas is important and the following are approved principles:*

1. *It is essential that no drops or no powder be instilled in the ear. No syringing should be done and no peroxide used.*
2. *If there is reason to suspect that the drum may be ruptured, but there is still some doubt because of blood or wax in the canal, leave the ear strictly alone.*
3. *The soldier should be warned to keep water out of the ear and avoid violent blowing of the nose.*
4. *A plug of sterile cotton should be placed in the canal and evacuation arranged to the nearest otologist.*[133]

The only exception to this is that a referral to an otolaryngologist is not urgent, because no additional treatment is appropriate for at least 3 months. Otolaryngologists generally wait 3 to 6 months for healing to occur before considering surgical repair.[132] There is good evidence that observation of tympanic membrane ruptures, with appropriate attention to preventing infection, provides superior healing compared with early surgical repair.[134]

EXTERNAL EAR
Otis Externa

Otitis externa (swimmer's ear, tropical ear) refers to inflammation of the external ear canal. It tends to present with first itching, then serous discharge, later pain (sometimes severe) and tenderness, particularly when the tragus is pressed (**Box 1**). Patients often complain of partial deafness from edema of the tympanic membrane, or mechanical blockage of the edematous external ear canal or from purulent drainage.

Otitis externa is more common in warm months in temperate climates, and in tropical or subtropical climates, likely related to increased humidity and sweating. Otitis externa occurs at all ages, although there is a bit of a peak from 7 to 12 years, and it tapers off after age 50.[135] Ten percent of people experience otitis externa at least once in their lives. Otitis externa is usually unilateral: only 10% of cases are bilateral.[108]

The external ear canal is protected by cerumen (ear wax). Cerumen is a combination of desquamated cells from the squamous epithelium of the external ear canal and secretions from glands in the canal. It is acidic and contains lysozyme, and it is thought to help prevent bacterial and fungal infection.[136,137] However, this has been recently challenged.[137,138]

Numerous factors are thought to predispose to otitis externa. Moisture in the external ear canal and a break in the normal protection of skin and cerumen (earwax)

> **Box 1**
> **Elements of the diagnosis of diffuse acute otitis externa**
>
> 1. Rapid onset (generally within 48 hours) in the past 3 weeks, AND
>
> 2. Symptoms of ear canal inflammation that include:
>
>   a. Otalgia (often severe), itching, or fullness,
>
>   b. WITH OR WITHOUT hearing loss or jaw pain,[a] AND
>
> 3. Signs of ear canal inflammation that include:
>
>   a. Tenderness of the tragus, pinna, or both
>
>   b. OR diffuse ear canal edema, erythema, or both
>
>   c. WITH OR WITHOUT otorrhea, regional lymphadenitis, tympanic membrane erythema, or cellulitis of the pinna and adjacent skin
>
> [a] Pain in the ear canal and temporomandibular joint region intensified by jaw motion.
> *From* Rosenfeld RM, Brown L, Cannon CR, et al. Clinical practice guideline: acute otitis externa. Otolaryngol Head Neck Surg 2006;134:S4-23; with permission.

are thought to be key. This is often a result of extended or repetitive swimming without drying the external ear canal afterward; from sweating profusely for a prolonged period; from hearing aids; or from the occlusive effect of earplugs or earbuds (in-ear speakers for mobile devices). Water in the external ear canal that is contaminated with large amounts of bacteria, or local trauma, perhaps from cleaning the canal with cotton swabs or other objects, is also thought to contribute.[139]

Otitis externa is classed into preinflammatory, acute inflammatory, and chronic stages. The preinflammatory stage is when dampness in the external ear canal causes swelling of the skin of the canal. This weakens the skin and obstructs glands that secrete cerumen. On examination with an otoscope, one sees the lining of the external ear canal turned whitish from the effects of moisture, and sometimes cerumen that is, rather than the characteristic medium yellow or brown, soft and quite pale, and sometimes whitish, again from the effects of moisture.[108]

On examining mild acute inflammatory otitis externa with an otoscope, one sees redness and mild swelling of the lining of the external ear canal, and perhaps some mild serous discharge. Moderate cases present with worsening pain, and on examination, one sees purulent discharge and enough edema that it is hard to see the tympanic membrane. Tenderness on pressing on the tragus or pulling on the pinna is a hallmark sign of otitis externa.[88] If the tympanic membrane is red, and there is suspicion of AOM, pneumatic otoscopy may show normal mobility, which rules out AOM.[88] Severe cases are so edematous, and with so much in the way of purulent discharge, that the lumen of the external ear canal is completely occluded, and the tympanic membrane is invisible. One may find swelling and redness even outside the external ear canal, visible without an otoscope, or adenopathy, particularly below and anterior to the ear. If the infection spreads to tissues outside the ear, particularly osteomyelitis of the temporal bone, this is termed malignant otitis externa (necrotizing otitis externa). Some say that "malignant" is a misnomer and "necrotizing" should be used instead because the process is infectious and not neoplastic.[140] Chronic otitis externa is defined by lasting more than a month, or recurring four or more times in 1 year.[136]

When because of severe otitis externa one is unable to see the tympanic membrane, it is hard to tell if one is dealing with isolated otitis externa or otitis media with tympanic rupture. However, the evidence suggests that appropriate treatment of moderate to severe otitis externa and of otitis media with a ruptured tympanic membrane are essentially the same.[88,141] To guide the topical antibiotic into the inner portion of the external ear canal, one may insert an expanding ear wick.[108]

A furuncle (abscess), an infected hair follicle, may appear in the outer third of the external ear canal. Pain and tenderness are focal, and as with any abscess, there may be purulent drainage, or, particularly in the era of MRSA, overlying cellulitis. This is sometimes termed focal otitis externa, but is a very different process from the more common otitis externa. Treatment is the same as for any abscess: local heat, and when clinically appropriate, incision and drainage; if there is significant overlying cellulitis, oral antibiotics that cover MRSA.[88]

Those who are immunocompromised (including diabetes mellitus) or who live in humid tropical environments are at risk for otomycosis, fungal infection of the outer ear. Drainage may be colorful: black, gray, bluish green, yellow, or white. Fungal hyphae may even be visible with an otoscope.[88,142]

The most common bacterium isolated from otitis externa is *P aeruginosa* (in roughly one-third of cases), *Staphylococcus epidermis* and *S aureus* (about 10% each), and a variety of other less-common bacteria in smaller frequencies. Fungi accounted for less than 2% (*Aspergillus* and *Candida*). *S epidermidis*, *Corynebacterium*, and α-hemolytic *Streptococcus* are normal flora, but may be implicated in infection when normal protective barriers in the external ear canal are breached.[135] Rare precipitants for otitis externa include infections from herpes simplex or varicella zoster virus (shingles) or eczema, which damage the squamous epithelium.[108]

Over the past two millennium a great variety of agents other than antibiotics have been used to treat otitis externa.[143,144] Steroids alone have been shown to be as effective as antibiotics.[102,103,145] Aluminum acetate, acetic acid, boric acid, and glycerine-ichthammol are all still used in the developing world, although good studies of their efficacy are not available except as described later.[146]

Because of its acid nature, vinegar has been used as a traditional medicine for infections, such as otitis externa, for thousands of years.[147] Two percent acetic acid has a pH of 3.[148] Commercial table vinegar, based on an inspection of a selection of material safety data sheets, has a pH of 2.2 to 2.6. Combinations of alcohol (for its drying effect) and acetic acid (or vinegar or lemon juice) to acidify, with or without hydrocortisone, have been traditionally used to prevent and treat otitis externa.[142] Prescription acetic acid drops with hydrocortisone (Vosol-HC, Actasol) or without hydrocortisone (Vosol, Acetasol) are available in the United States. These are probably effective for mild cases; however, they may be painful to an irritated ear canal, must be used multiple times a day, and should not be used with tympanostomy tubes or a tympanic membrane perforation because there are concerns about ototoxicity of acetic acid.[149]

In vitro studies show that aluminum acetate and acetic acid are effective against common bacteria causing otitis externa.[150] One study showed aluminum acetate drops clinically effective in chronic otitis with otorrhea (including those with perforated tympanic membranes).[151] Aluminum acetate is available quite inexpensively over-the-counter as Burow Solution (13% aluminum acetate; domeboro) with a pH of 3.06.

Given their high concentrations and persistence and lack of systemic side effects, and concerns about rising antibiotic resistance, a consensus panel recommends that ear drops should be used instead of systemic antibiotics as the primary treatment of otitis externa and otorrhea with tympanostomy tubes.[152] Oral antibiotics may be added to ear drops (not substituted for ear drops) when the patient is immunocompromised by such conditions as diabetes mellitus, local radiotherapy, or HIV-AIDS, or when the infection extends outside the ear canal (malignant otitis externa).[88,142] There is some evidence that treating otitis externa with common antibiotics used for AOM actually interferes with resolution of the otitis externa and, in the case of cephalosporins, increases recurrence rates.[88]

The natural history of otitis externa shows that without treatment, only 15% of patients experience a clinical cure at 10 days. Antimicrobial ear drops, whether antiseptic or antibiotic (or, surprisingly, steroid drops alone), are highly effective, raising this 10-day cure rate to 65% to 80%.[153]

A combination of the aminoglycoside neomycin with the polypeptide antibiotic polymyxin, for additional coverage of *P aeruginosa*, and hydrocortisone, to decrease swelling (Cortisporin) is quite commonly prescribed. However, neomycin is well-known to dermatologists as a common skin allergen,[154–156] which may complicate the otitis externa with a severe local reaction, making these drops undesirable as a first-line treatment of otitis externa. If one is seeing a patient with persistent or worsening otitis externa despite being on neomycin drops, changing to a quinolone antibiotic combined with a steroid is appropriate. Seeing a pattern of eczematous eruption on the lower portion of the external ear where ear drops tend to run may be a clue to such an allergic reaction.[142] Ten percent to 15% of the normal population is hypersensitive to neomycin.[88]

Neomycin is also an aminoglycoside, and aminoglycosides are considered ototoxic.[98,99] They should only be used in cases of potential tympanic membrane perforation (eg, severe otitis externa where the tympanic membrane cannot be visualized) or when there are tympanostomy tubes when the benefits clearly outweigh the risks.

Topical fluoroquinolones first became available to treat otitis externa in 1997 and 1998 in the form of ciprofloxacin and ofloxacin. With excellent coverage of gram-positive and -negative bacteria including *P aeruginosa*, and without the ototoxicity or allergy concerns of neomycin,[157,158] quinolones seem an ideal antibiotic for otitis externa. In addition to ciprofloxacin (Ciprodex, Cipro-HC), ofloxacin ear drops (Floxin) are available. These have been specifically studied in one study of hundreds of patients and found to be more effective than prior treatments and safe with tympanostomy tubes (and, by a reasonable extension, in those with ruptured tympanic membranes).[159] Multiple studies have shown that ciprofloxacin (with or without hydrocortisone or dexamethasone) and ofloxacin drops are as effective as neomycin-polymyxin-hydrocortisone ear drops.[160–163] In one study, once-daily ofloxacin ear drops were as effective as neomycin-polymyxin-hydrocortisone ear drops four times a day.[157] Beers and Abramo[108] pointed out that ciprofloxacin-hydrocortisone ear drops had not been studied for safety in the setting of tympanostomy tubes or a ruptured tympanic membrane, and thus recommended ofloxacin ear drops for this particular setting. However, there seems to be no solid evidence for ototoxicity of the combination of ciprofloxacin and dexamethasone, and there is now literature that suggests its use in otorrhea with tympanostomy tubes is safe and effective, and may be more effective than ofloxacin.[158] Ciprofloxacin and particularly ofloxacin have some activity against MRSA,[164–166] and quinolone antibiotics stay at very high concentrations in the external ear, making efficacy against MRSA and even quinolone-resistant *S aureus* quite likely; quinolone ear drops also have no significant systemic absorption, making emergence of ciprofloxacin resistance unlikely.[149]

The evidence seems to favor ofloxacin (Floxin) or ciprofloxacin-dexamethasone (Ciprodex) drops as the first choice for treating otitis externa or otorrhea with tubes (and by a reasonable generalization, AOM with tympanic rupture), and once-a-day dosing of ofloxacin is likely appropriate.[167] Cost of quinolone antibiotic ear drops used to be a major concern (on the order of $100 per prescription). However, inexpensive generic ofloxacin ear drops are now available; for example, the MedExpress chain of urgent care centers currently (2012) charges patients $15 for a bottle, and the Massachusetts Department of Health currently lists it having a charge of $10.92. There are recommendations against using benzocaine-containing analgesic ear drops for otitis externa (eg, Auralgan), given the concerns for potential allergic reactions to the benzocaine complicating ongoing assessment of the efficacy of treatment.[88]

The technique for instilling ear drops may make a significant difference in how they work. When prescribing ear drops for otitis externa, gently cleanse secretions and wax out of the ear. Instruct the patient to gently cleanse the ear at home before instilling the drops. Warm the ear drops to body temperature, perhaps by keeping in a shirt or pants pocket for 5 to 10 minutes before use. This prevents dizziness from caloric stimulation (difference in temperature causing circulation in the semicircular canal). Have the patient lie on the unaffected side; instill the drops (gently pulling on the pinna may open the ear canal a bit to allow the drops in); and then gently press on the tragus a few times to pump the drops deeper into the ear. Have the patient stay lying on the side for a few minutes after instilling. Placing a cotton ball in the ear before arising may prevent the drops from draining out of the ear onto the patient's clothes; this may be removed after the danger of such external drainage has ceased.[142]

Patients with otitis externa should be instructed to abstain from water sports for 7 to 10 days after treatment starts. Competitive swimmers may return to swimming 2 to 3 days after treatment, or immediately if they wear well-fitting ear plugs after the pain has resolved. Hearing aids and ear buds (in-ear speakers) should remain out until pain and discharge have resolved.[88]

Patients should be told to expect a significant improvement in their pain and discharge in 2 to 3 days. If not improving by then, patients should be instructed to have their ears reassessed. The possibility of AOM with ruptured tympanic membrane may be entertained, and if there is ongoing pain or fever, an appropriate oral antibiotic for AOM might be appropriate. The patient must be reassessed for the possibility of malignant otitis media (see next). The ear may need to be cleaned of debris to ensure that the topical antibiotic is delivered to the entire ear canal. This may require IV analgesia or even moderate sedation. A culture for bacterial and fungal pathogens is appropriate. It may also be necessary to consult an otolaryngologist for urgent follow-up, because failure to improve may be an indication of something other than simple otitis externa, such as cancer.[88]

Malignant Otitis Externa

Malignant otitis externa is primarily a problem of those with immunosuppression, most commonly from diabetes mellitus or HIV-AIDS. The mortality of 50% before antibiotics is now much lower, estimated to be 0% to 15%. Examination of the ear canal may show exposed bone or granulation tissue, particularly in the inferior portion of the canal, although the tympanic membrane usually appears normal. Pain out of proportion to examination findings, history of immunosuppression, and an elevated erythrocyte sedimentation rate in the face of normal temperature and white blood cell count tend to suggest malignant otitis externa. MRI is superior to CT in confirming the diagnosis, and may show dural enhancement and involvement of medullary bone spaces. However, a technetium or gallium scan is the preferred diagnostic test, although it is positive in other local inflammatory conditions, including cancer. A culture of the exudate should be sent before IV antibiotics are started. Because carcinoma and other conditions may present similarly, a biopsy is usually performed.[140]

It has been shown that cerumen in diabetic ears has an alkaline pH rather than a normal acidic pH, and this may be one of the reasons why malignant otitis externa is most common in people with diabetes (65%–90% of cases). Elderly people with diabetes also tend to have endarteritis, microangiopathy, and small vessel oblitera-tion, which is thought to contribute.[168] The ability of *P aeruginosa* to invade tissues and cause septic thrombophlebitis makes it by far the most common bacterium impli-cated in malignant otitis externa. It is considered an opportunistic pathogen.[169] Fungi, such as *Aspergillus*, are uncommon as a cause of malignant otitis externa except in patients with HIV with CD4 counts less than 50 cells/mm^3.[169]

Complications of malignant otitis externa include damage to the facial nerve, necrosis of the tympanic membrane, stenosis of the external ear canal (EAC), auricular deformity, and sensorineural and conductive hearing loss. Treatment consists of several weeks of IV antibiotics; in children, fluoroquinolones are used only if the bene-fits outweigh the risks of joint damage. Given the increasing resistance of *P aeruginosa* to fluoroquinolones, antipseudomonal penicillins and cephalosporins are now gener-ally the treatment of choice combined with an antibiotic appropriate for MRSA until cultures are available.[88,140] Rare cases of malignant otitis externa caused by the fungus *Aspergillus* are treated with IV antifungals.[170]

Cholesteatoma

Cholesteatomas are epidermal inclusion cysts of the middle ear or mastoid. Early investigators thought these "pearly tumors" contained cholesterol crystals[171] but it is now known that they are filled with desquamated keratinaceous material, similar to the "sebaceous" epidermal cysts found on the skin. As with epidermal cysts of the skin, they may become infected, causing drainage. Cholesteatomas may also, by either direct extension or becoming infected, result in bone destruction or even intracranial infection. Frequently they may become infected with anaerobic bacteria, resulting in otorrhea with a characteristic and almost feculent odor.[172] Cholesteato-mas may also present with a variety of symptoms, depending on the location and extent: vertigo, hearing loss, facial nerve paralysis, or intracranial infection. The classic location for a cholesteatoma is adjacent to the posterosuperior portion of the tympanic membrane, but they may appear in other portions of the external ear canal, or perfo-rating through the tympanic membrane.[173]

If infected, cholesteatomas should be treated with appropriate topical antibiotics. If suspicious of osteomyelitis, CT or MRI is appropriate; as with any suspected infection or tumor, IV contrast improves the diagnostic quality of CT and MRI. Patients with cho-lesteatomas should generally be referred to an otolaryngologist for ongoing care.

Perichondritis

Perichondritis of the ear, specifically infectious perichondritis, is becoming more common because of the popularity of piercing of the upper portion of the pinna. Piercing of the upper portion of the ear, through the less infection-resistant cartilage, exposes those subjected to it to a higher likelihood of more serious infections, but this seems to be widely unknown by those performing or receiving such piercings. The goals of treatment include healing without permanent deformity. *P aeruginosa* and *S aureus* are common pathogens. Surgical drainage is sometimes required, and systemic antibiotic coverage for both of the previously mentioned pathogens is recommended.[174]

CERUMEN IMPACTION

A 2008 American Academy of Otolaryngology–Head and Neck Surgery Foundation clinical practice guideline[175] is currently the definitive reference for managing cerumen impactions. The following represents a distillation of the portions of this guideline relevant to the practice of emergency medicine.

Cerumen impaction (defined by the 2008 clinical guideline as either complete or partial occlusion of the external ear canal with excess cerumen) is found in 1 of every 10 children, 1 of every 20 adults, in a third of the elderly, and in a third of those with developmental delay. If asymptomatic, cerumen need not be removed. However, cerumen impaction may diminish cognitive function in the elderly, and may interfere with visualization of the tympanic membrane during otoscopy. Cerumen impaction may also cause hearing loss, tinnitus, vertigo, fullness, itching, otalgia, discharge, odor, or cough; however, these may be a symptom of another process coincident with cerumen impaction. Cerumen removal may help achieve a diagnosis, either by relieving the symptoms or by allowing visualization of the external ear canal and tympanic membrane.

Cerumen removal has risks and benefits; it may result in external ear canal pain, abrasions or lacerations, vertigo, syncope, or otitis externa. Tympanic membrane perforation or hearing loss are rare complications. However, one study showed a 0.2% incidence of tympanic membrane perforation from irrigation, and a similar 0.2% incidence of vertigo. One should also consider confounding conditions that might change one's choice of methods for cerumen removal, such as nonintact tympanic membrane (perforation or tympanostomy tube); ear canal stenosis; exostoses; diabetes mellitus; immunocompromised state; or anticoagulant therapy.

In some of these cases, safe removal in the emergency department may not be possible, and cerumen removal may have to be deferred, to be performed later by an otolaryngologist using a binocular microscope and microinstrumentation. There are three main methods used to remove cerumen: (1) cerumenolytic agents; (2) irrigation; and (3) manual removal, using ear curettes, probes, hooks, forceps, or microsuction. There is no evidence as to which of these, or which combination of them, is best.

There is some evidence that cerumenolytic agents may aid in removal of cerumen, but no evidence that any one agent is superior to the others. The guideline recommends that cerumenolytic agents not be used in patients with otitis externa, because otitis externa is an exclusion for studies of such agents. There are also concerns about a reported 1% skin allergy incidence to 10% triethanolamine polypeptide oleate (Cerumenex) drops. There is some evidence that cerumenolytic agents used before irrigation may improve the efficacy of irrigation. Even water or normal saline used as a cerumenolytic drop 15 minutes before irrigation improved efficacy.

When the tympanic membrane is not intact, mechanical removal might be attempted in the emergency department, but irrigation should be avoided because of concerns about pain, infection, caloric vertigo, and ototoxic hearing loss.

Atrophy of the tympanic membrane from prior surgery, including tympanostomy tubes, is a risk for tympanic membrane rupture, so irrigation is not recommended for those who have had such surgery in the past. When the patient is immunocompromised, for example by diabetes mellitus or HIV-AIDS, concerns about causing malignant otitis externa should prevent routine tap water irrigation unless great care is taken to avoid abrasions, and one considers prescribing acidifying ear drops, such as 2% acetic acid (Vosol, Acetasol) two drops in each ear twice a day, or recommending over-the-counter drops, such as aluminum acetate (Burow solution, Domeboro).

Mechanical removal of cerumen may be faster than irrigation; allows a direct view of the external ear canal; and does not make the external ear canal wet, which is thought to be a risk for otitis externa. Mechanical removal is preferred over irrigation or cerumenolytic agents for patients with a nonintact tympanic membrane or the potential for it, or prior ear surgery. Manual removal, with or without cerumenolytic agents, is preferred over irrigation for those with immunosuppression caused by such conditions as diabetes mellitus or HIV-AIDS, or who may be immunosuppressed because of systemic illness.

There are many devices available for mechanical removal of cerumen. Perhaps the most effective tool is the binocular microscope often used by otolaryngologists, which is seldom available in the emergency department; those with abnormal external ear canals may benefit from a referral to an otolaryngologist for removal using such a device. Barring such abnormalities, removal in the emergency department under direct visualization with the combination of a headlight, an otoscope speculum, and either a metal or plastic curette may be effective. Those who are on anticoagulants should have cerumen removed by instrumentation only with the greatest care, and the use of cerumenolytics and irrigation may be a better option for them.

There are consensus opinions that certain methods of home removal are not appropriate. These include the use of oral jet irrigators, which may cause ear trauma, and cotton-tip swabs, which may also cause ear trauma, including a ruptured tympanic membrane. There is even a case report of a fatal brain abscess from retained cotton in the ear.

Those with dermatologic diseases of the ear canal, recurrent otitis externa, keratosis obturans, prior radiation therapy affecting the ear, previous tympanoplasty or myringoplasty, or canal wall down mastoidectomy should have their cerumen impactions managed by an otolaryngologist.

Patients with cerumen impactions may be counseled on recommended home care. This includes not using bobby pins or cotton swabs to attempt to remove wax, because this may traumatize the ear and tends to pack cerumen up against the tympanic membrane. Weekly use of a topical ear emollient may significantly (61% vs 23%) decrease future cerumen impactions.

FOREIGN BODIES IN EARS

Foreign body in the ear is a common presentation to primary care offices, emergency departments, and urgent care centers. However, there is little literature on the topic except for case reports and case reviews, and there are no controlled studies to allow one to conclude that one method is superior, either in terms of efficacy or in terms of complications, such as tympanic membrane perforation or external ear canal laceration. Therefore, the following provides an overview of the literature and expert opinion expressed in this literature.

One retrospective case review, which focused solely on those patients referred to otolaryngologists, and thus does not likely reflect most cases, found that about half of those cases referred to an ear, nose, and throat physician after attempted removal by an emergency physician or primary care physician had lacerations of the external canal; however, there is no information on the corresponding number of foreign bodies that were successfully removed by an emergency physician or primary care physician. The article also notes that otolaryngologists tend to use a microscope to remove foreign bodies (91% of the time).[176] The most common foreign body in this study was a cockroach (43 of 98) followed by beads (15 of 98). The study recommends lidocaine instillation (provided the tympanic membrane is intact), which in their series rather than paralyzing the cockroaches, caused them to quickly back out. The recommendations from this case series are as follows:

- Preremoval hearing assessment for patients in who damage to the hearing is suspected
- Removal under direct vision, using a microscope if appropriate

- Patients with objects not readily removed by the primary care physician may require referral to an otolaryngologist
- Mineral oil or lidocaine aural instillation may be useful adjuncts during the removal of live cockroaches

A prospective review from an otolaryngology service in Brazil found that beans were the most common foreign body in the ear.[177] A different retrospective review of 141 cases presenting to primary care offices and the emergency department of an eye and ear hospital found cockroaches to be less common ("insects" 21 of 141), and beads (31 of 141), plastic toys (29 of 141), and pebbles (21 of 141) to be the most common. This study mentioned common instruments available for removal: Frazier tip suctions, alligator forceps, Hartman forceps, cerumen loops, and right-angle ball hooks.

Right-angle ball hooks have a thin (few millimeter) rod that makes a right angle at the end, with a blunted end, sufficient to slip into the central hole of a bead. These have been improvised by straightening and then bending the very tip of a paper clip; this has the disadvantage that it is not smooth at the tip, which makes it harder to slip into the hold in the bead. The paper also mentions the Schuknecht foreign body remover, a commercially available 22-gauge angled suction catheter. This study makes a recommendation to avoid any attempts at irrigation if the foreign body could be a small button battery, because of the possibility of damage from short-circuiting the battery with resultant burns to the ear. It goes on to make specific recommendations for referral to an otolaryngologist:

- Lack of proper instrumentation
- Lack of staff to adequately restrain uncooperative child
- Failure to remove foreign body on initial attempts
- Existent injury to the external auditory canal or tympanic membrane
- Object wedged in the medial external auditory canal or up against tympanic membrane
- Glass or other sharp-edged foreign body
- Special circumstances, such as insects, putty, and disk batteries

One retrospective pediatric emergency department study found only 4 of 58 ear foreign bodies were successfully removed in their Australian emergency department.[178] Another pediatric emergency department study, a retrospective chart review of 36 cases over a 1-year period, found a better success ratio (53%) but found a higher complication rate in rounded objects that were hard to grasp, and concluded "certain foreign bodies (graspable type) of the EAC in pediatric patients can be successfully managed by skilled emergency department personnel with low complication rates, whereas other foreign bodies (nongraspable types) may be better managed by early referral to an otolaryngologist."[179]

A literature review from 2000 notes that the literature frequently recommends restraining children before attempts at removal, but that modern emergency medicine capability makes moderate sedation a more humane option. It also notes that irrigation is contraindicated if there is a tympanostomy tube or ruptured tympanic membrane, or if there is vegetable matter that may swell.[180]

A variety of methods have been reported successful in isolated case reports to remove foreign bodies from the ear, and a listing of these might make one more likely to find a method appropriate for a particular instance. These include the following:

- Killing an insect with vinegar then removing with a probe (recommendation from the era of the Roman Empire)[180]

- Binding the patient to a table with the affected ear down and then pounding on the table (another Roman recommendation)[180]
- Cyanoacrylate glue on the end of an instrument to remove a bead[181]
- A Jobson Horne probe (a steel probe with a circle of steel on the end, used sometimes for removing cerumen) or steel wire loop[180]
- Impression materials: pouring a fast-setting flexible material into the ear canal, and then removing the resulting plug including the foreign body[182]
- A paper clip bent into an appropriately shaped loop[182,183]
- Tiny magnets[184]
- Using ethyl chloride to dissolve Styrofoam beads[185]

Sticking a hollow candle in the ear and lighting it is a traditional "holistic" remedy for a variety of ear conditions, including the impacted cerumen. It does not remove cerumen, and causes many complications, including occlusions of the external ear canal with candle wax, tympanic perforation, otitis externa, and burns of the auricle. There are strong recommendations in the medical literature that ear candles should never be used by anyone for any reason whatsoever.[175,186,187]

REFERENCES

1. Teele DW, Klein JO, Rosner B. Epidemiology of otitis media during the first seven years of life in children in greater Boston: a prospective, cohort study. J Infect Dis 1989;160:83–94.
2. Schappert SM. Office visits for otitis media: United States, 1975-90. Adv Data 1992;(214):1–19.
3. Stool SE, Field MJ. The impact of otitis media. Pediatr Infect Dis J 1989;8:S11–4.
4. Grijalva CG, Poehling KA, Nuorti JP, et al. National impact of universal childhood immunization with pneumococcal conjugate vaccine on outpatient medical care visits in the United States. Pediatrics 2006;118:865–73.
5. Stamboulidis K, Chatzaki D, Poulakou G, et al. The impact of the heptavalent pneumococcal conjugate vaccine on the epidemiology of acute otitis media complicated by otorrhea. Pediatr Infect Dis J 2011;30:551–5.
6. Fisher EW, Parikh AA, Harcourt JP, et al. The burden of screening for acoustic neuroma: asymmetric otological symptoms in the ENT clinic. Clin Otolaryngol Allied Sci 1994;19:19–21.
7. Wiener SL. Differential diagnosis of acute pain: by body region. New York: McGraw-Hill; 1993.
8. Leonetti JP, Li J, Smith PG. Otalgia. An isolated symptom of malignant infratemporal tumors. Am J Otol 1998;19:496–8.
9. Ely JW, Hansen MR, Clark EC. Diagnosis of ear pain. Am Fam Physician 2008; 77:621–8.
10. Fliss DM, Leiberman A, Dagan R. Medical sequelae and complications of acute otitis media. Pediatr Infect Dis J 1994;13:S34–40 [discussion: S50–4].
11. Hendley JO. Clinical practice. Otitis media. N Engl J Med 2002;347:1169–74.
12. Dowell SF, Marcy SM, Phillips WR, et al. Otitis media—principles of judicious use of antimicrobial agents. Pediatrics 1998;101:165–71.
13. Hayden GF. Acute suppurative otitis media in children. Diversity of clinical diagnostic criteria. Clin Pediatr (Phila) 1981;20:99–104.
14. Finitzo T, Friel-Patti S, Chinn K, et al. Tympanometry and otoscopy prior to myringotomy: issues in diagnosis of otitis media. Int J Pediatr Otorhinolaryngol 1992;24:101–10.

15. Rosenfeld RM, Culpepper L, Doyle KJ, et al. Clinical practice guideline: otitis media with effusion. Otolaryngol Head Neck Surg 2004;130:S95–118.
16. Weiss JC, Yates GR, Quinn LD. Acute otitis media: making an accurate diagnosis. Am Fam Physician 1996;53:1200–6.
17. Chianese J, Hoberman A, Paradise JL, et al. Spectral gradient acoustic reflectometry compared with tympanometry in diagnosing middle ear effusion in children aged 6 to 24 months. Arch Pediatr Adolesc Med 2007;161:884–8.
18. Pelton SI. Otoscopy for the diagnosis of otitis media. Pediatr Infect Dis J 1998; 17:540–3 [discussion: 80].
19. Popelka GR. Acoustic immittance measures: terminology and instrumentation. Ear Hear 1984;5:262–7.
20. Tympanometry. ASHA Working Group on Aural Acoustic-Immittance Measurements Committee on Audiologic Evaluation. J Speech Hear Disord 1988;53: 354–77.
21. Kimball S. Acoustic reflectometry: spectral gradient analysis for improved detection of middle ear effusion in children. Pediatr Infect Dis J 1998;17: 552–5 [discussion: 80].
22. Stewart MH, Siff JE, Cydulka RK. Evaluation of the patient with sore throat, earache, and sinusitis: an evidence based approach. Emerg Med Clin North Am 1999;17:153–87, ix.
23. Laine MK, Tahtinen PA, Helenius KK, et al. Acoustic reflectometry in discrimination of otoscopic diagnoses in young ambulatory children. Pediatr Infect Dis J 2012;31:1007–11.
24. Teppo H, Revonta M. Comparison of old, professional and consumer model acoustic reflectometers in the detection of middle-ear fluid in children with recurrent acute otitis media or glue ear. Int J Pediatr Otorhinolaryngol 2007;71: 1865–72.
25. Combs JT. The diagnosis of otitis media: new techniques. Pediatr Infect Dis J 1994;13:1039–46.
26. Kontiokari T, Koivunen P, Niemela M, et al. Symptoms of acute otitis media. Pediatr Infect Dis J 1998;17:676–9.
27. Del Mar C, Glasziou P, Hayem M. Are antibiotics indicated as initial treatment for children with acute otitis media? A meta-analysis. BMJ 1997;314:1526–9.
28. Van Zuijlen DA, Schilder AG, Van Balen FA, et al. National differences in incidence of acute mastoiditis: relationship to prescribing patterns of antibiotics for acute otitis media? Pediatr Infect Dis J 2001;20:140–4.
29. Akkerman AE, Kuyvenhoven MM, van der Wouden JC, et al. Analysis of under- and overprescribing of antibiotics in acute otitis media in general practice. J Antimicrob Chemother 2005;56:569–74.
30. Froom J, Culpepper L, Grob P, et al. Diagnosis and antibiotic treatment of acute otitis media: report from International Primary Care Network. BMJ 1990;300: 582–6.
31. Froom J, Culpepper L, Green LA, et al. A cross-national study of acute otitis media: risk factors, severity, and treatment at initial visit. Report from the International Primary Care Network (IPCN) and the Ambulatory Sentinel Practice Network (ASPN). J Am Board Fam Pract 2001;14:406–17.
32. Berman S. Otitis media in developing countries. Pediatrics 1995;96:126–31.
33. Acuin J. Chronic suppurative otitis media: burden of illness and management options. Geneva (Switzerland): World Health Organization; 2004.
34. Davidson J, Hyde ML, Alberti PW. Epidemiologic patterns in childhood hearing loss: a review. Int J Pediatr Otorhinolaryngol 1989;17:239–66.

35. Bluestone CD. Otitis media in children: to treat or not to treat? N Engl J Med 1982;306:1399–404.
36. Cates C. An evidence based approach to reducing antibiotic use in children with acute otitis media: controlled before and after study. BMJ 1999;318:715–6.
37. Siegel RM, Kiely M, Bien JP, et al. Treatment of otitis media with observation and a safety-net antibiotic prescription. Pediatrics 2003;112:527–31.
38. Chao JH, Kunkov S, Reyes LB, et al. Comparison of two approaches to observation therapy for acute otitis media in the emergency department. Pediatrics 2008;121:e1352–6.
39. McCormick DP, Chonmaitree T, Pittman C, et al. Nonsevere acute otitis media: a clinical trial comparing outcomes of watchful waiting versus immediate antibiotic treatment. Pediatrics 2005;115:1455–65.
40. Little P, Gould C, Williamson I, et al. Pragmatic randomised controlled trial of two prescribing strategies for childhood acute otitis media. BMJ 2001;322:336–42.
41. Hoberman A, Paradise JL, Rockette HE, et al. Treatment of acute otitis media in children under 2 years of age. N Engl J Med 2011;364:105–15.
42. Damoiseaux RA, van Balen FA, Hoes AW, et al. Antibiotic treatment of acute otitis media in children under two years of age: evidence based? Br J Gen Pract 1998;48:1861–4.
43. Glasziou PP, Del Mar CB, Sanders SL, et al. Antibiotics for acute otitis media in children. Cochrane Database Syst Rev 2004;(1):CD000219.
44. Klein JO. Children under 2 years of age with acute otitis media benefit from antibiotic treatment. J Pediatr 2011;159:514–5.
45. Rovers MM, Glasziou P, Appelman CL, et al. Antibiotics for acute otitis media: a meta-analysis with individual patient data. Lancet 2006;368:1429–35.
46. Rovers MM, Glasziou P, Appelman CL, et al. Predictors of pain and/or fever at 3 to 7 days for children with acute otitis media not treated initially with antibiotics: a meta-analysis of individual patient data. Pediatrics 2007;119:579–85.
47. Marchant CD, Carlin SA, Johnson CE, et al. Measuring the comparative efficacy of antibacterial agents for acute otitis media: the "Pollyanna phenomenon". J Pediatr 1992;120:72–7.
48. Damoiseaux RA, van Balen FA, Hoes AW, et al. Primary care based randomised, double blind trial of amoxicillin versus placebo for acute otitis media in children aged under 2 years. BMJ 2000;320:350–4.
49. Vergison A, Dagan R, Arguedas A, et al. Otitis media and its consequences: beyond the earache. Lancet Infect Dis 2010;10:195–203.
50. American Academy of Pediatrics Subcommittee on Management of Acute Otitis Media. Diagnosis and management of acute otitis media. Pediatrics 2004;113:1451–65.
51. Vernacchio L, Vezina RM, Mitchell AA. Management of acute otitis media by primary care physicians: trends since the release of the 2004 American Academy of Pediatrics/American Academy of Family Physicians clinical practice guideline. Pediatrics 2007;120:281–7.
52. Coco A, Vernacchio L, Horst M, et al. Management of acute otitis media after publication of the 2004 AAP and AAFP clinical practice guideline. Pediatrics 2010;125:214–20.
53. Sanders SL, Glasziou PP, Del Mar CB, et al. Antibiotics for acute otitis media in children. Cochrane Database Syst Rev 2010;(4):CD000219.
54. Takata GS, Chan LS, Shekelle P, et al. Evidence assessment of management of acute otitis media: I. The role of antibiotics in treatment of uncomplicated acute otitis media. Pediatrics 2001;108:239–47.

55. Thanaviratananich S, Laopaiboon M, Vatanasapt P. Once or twice daily versus three times daily amoxicillin with or without clavulanate for the treatment of acute otitis media. Cochrane Database of Systematic Reviews. Chichester (United Kingdom): John Wiley & Sons, Ltd; 2008.

56. Kozyrskyj A, Klassen TP, Moffatt M, et al. Short-course antibiotics for acute otitis media. Cochrane Database Syst Rev 2010;(9):CD001095.

57. Dowell SF, Butler JC, Giebink GS, et al. Acute otitis media: management and surveillance in an era of pneumococcal resistance: a report from the Drug-resistant *Streptococcus pneumoniae* Therapeutic Working Group. Pediatr Infect Dis J 1999;18:1–9.

58. Leibovitz E, Greenberg D, Piglansky L, et al. Recurrent acute otitis media occurring within one month from completion of antibiotic therapy: relationship to the original pathogen. Pediatr Infect Dis J 2003;22:209–16.

59. Harsten G, Prellner K, Heldrup J, et al. Recurrent acute otitis media. A prospective study of children during the first three years of life. Acta Otolaryngol 1989; 107:111–9.

60. Alho OP, Laara E, Oja H. What is the natural history of recurrent acute otitis media in infancy? J Fam Pract 1996;43:258–64.

61. Berman S. Otitis media in children. N Engl J Med 1995;332:1560–5.

62. Coleman C, Moore M. Decongestants and antihistamines for acute otitis media in children. Cochrane Database Syst Rev 2007;(2):CD001727.

63. Eyibilen A, Aladag I, Guven M, et al. The effectiveness of nasal decongestants, oral decongestants and oral decongestant-antihistamines in the treatment of acute otitis media in children. Kulak Burun Bogaz Ihtis Derg 2009;19:289–93.

64. Randall JE, Hendley JO. A decongestant-antihistamine mixture in the prevention of otitis media in children with colds. Pediatrics 1979;63:483–5.

65. Taverner D, Latte GJ. Nasal decongestants for the common cold. Cochrane Database of Systematic Reviews. Chichester (United Kingdom): John Wiley & Sons, Ltd; 2009.

66. Eccles R, Martensson K, Chen SC. Effects of intranasal xylometazoline, alone or in combination with ipratropium, in patients with common cold. Curr Med Res Opin 2010;26(4):889–99.

67. Hoberman A, Paradise JL, Reynolds EA, et al. Efficacy of Auralgan for treating ear pain in children with acute otitis media. Arch Pediatr Adolesc Med 1997;151: 675–8.

68. Foxlee R, Johansson A, Wejfalk J, et al. Topical analgesia for acute otitis media. Cochrane Database Syst Rev 2006;(3):CD005657.

69. Bodor FF, Marchant CD, Shurin PA, et al. Bacterial etiology of conjunctivitis-otitis media syndrome. Pediatrics 1985;76:26–8.

70. Bingen E, Cohen R, Jourenkova N, et al. Epidemiologic study of conjunctivitis-otitis syndrome. Pediatr Infect Dis J 2005;24:731–2.

71. Bodor FF. Systemic antibiotics for treatment of the conjunctivitis-otitis media syndrome. Pediatr Infect Dis J 1989;8:287–90.

72. Harrison CJ, Hedrick JA, Block SL, et al. Relation of the outcome of conjunctivitis and the conjunctivitis-otitis syndrome to identifiable risk factors and oral antimicrobial therapy. Pediatr Infect Dis J 1987;6:536–40.

73. Gigliotti F, Williams WT, Hayden FG, et al. Etiology of acute conjunctivitis in children. J Pediatr 1981;98:531–6.

74. Gilbert DN. The Sanford guide to antimicrobial therapy 2011. Sperryville (VA): Antimicrobial Therapy, Inc; 2011.

75. Bodor FF. Conjunctivitis-otitis syndrome. Pediatrics 1982;69:695–8.

76. Nelson JD, Ginsburg CM, McLeland O, et al. Concentrations of antimicrobial agents in middle ear fluid, saliva and tears. Int J Pediatr Otorhinolaryngol 1981;3:327–34.

77. Teele DW, Klein JO, Rosner BA. Epidemiology of otitis media in children. Ann Otol Rhinol Laryngol Suppl 1980;89:5–6.

78. Bluestone CD. Eustachian tube function and allergy in otitis media. Pediatrics 1978;61:753–60.

79. Bluestone CD, Hebda PA, Alper CM, et al. Recent advances in otitis media. 2. Eustachian tube, middle ear, and mastoid anatomy; physiology, pathophysiology, and pathogenesis. Ann Otol Rhinol Laryngol Suppl 2005;194:16–30.

80. Klein JO. Otitis media. Clin Infect Dis 1994;19:823–33.

81. Perera R, Haynes J, Glasziou P, et al. Autoinflation for hearing loss associated with otitis media with effusion. Cochrane Database Syst Rev 2006;(4):CD006285.

82. Simpson SA, Lewis R, van der Voort J, et al. Oral or topical nasal steroids for hearing loss associated with otitis media with effusion in children. Cochrane Database Syst Rev 2011;(5):CD001935.

83. van Zon A, van der Heijden GJ, van Dongen TM, et al. Antibiotics for otitis media with effusion in children. Cochrane Database Syst Rev 2012;(9):CD009163.

84. Griffin G, Flynn CA. Antihistamines and/or decongestants for otitis media with effusion (OME) in children. Cochrane Database Syst Rev 2011;(9):CD003423.

85. van der Merwe J, Wagenfeld DJ. The negative effects of mucolytics in otitis media with effusion. S Afr Med J 1987;72:625–6.

86. Finkelstein Y, Ophir D, Talmi YP, et al. Adult-onset otitis media with effusion. Arch Otolaryngol Head Neck Surg 1994;120:517–27.

87. Bernstein JM. Role of allergy in eustachian tube blockage and otitis media with effusion: a review. Otolaryngol Head Neck Surg 1996;114:562–8.

88. Rosenfeld RM, Brown L, Cannon CR, et al. Clinical practice guideline: acute otitis externa. Otolaryngol Head Neck Surg 2006;134:S4–23.

89. McLelland CA. Incidence of complications from use of tympanostomy tubes. Arch Otolaryngol 1980;106:97–9.

90. Gates GA, Avery C, Prihoda TJ, et al. Delayed onset post-tympanotomy otorrhea. Otolaryngol Head Neck Surg 1988;98:111–5.

91. Berger G. Nature of spontaneous tympanic membrane perforation in acute otitis media in children. J Laryngol Otol 1989;103:1150–3.

92. Granath A, Rynnel-Dagoo B, Backheden M, et al. Tube associated otorrhea in children with recurrent acute otitis media; results of a prospective randomized study on bacteriology and topical treatment with or without systemic antibiotics. Int J Pediatr Otorhinolaryngol 2008;72:1225–33.

93. Ruohola A, Meurman O, Nikkari S, et al. Microbiology of acute otitis media in children with tympanostomy tubes: prevalences of bacteria and viruses. Clin Infect Dis 2006;43:1417–22.

94. Mandel EM, Casselbrant ML, Kurs-Lasky M. Acute otorrhea: bacteriology of a common complication of tympanostomy tubes. Ann Otol Rhinol Laryngol 1994;103:713–8.

95. Goldblatt EL. Efficacy of ofloxacin and other otic preparations for acute otitis media in patients with tympanostomy tubes. Pediatr Infect Dis J 2001;20: 116–9 [discussion: 20–2].

96. Roland PS, Parry DA, Stroman DW. Microbiology of acute otitis media with tympanostomy tubes. Otolaryngol Head Neck Surg 2005;133:585–95.

97. Saunders MW, Robinson PJ. How easily do topical antibiotics pass through tympanostomy tubes? An in vitro study. Int J Pediatr Otorhinolaryngol 1999;50:45–50.

98. Wright CG, Meyerhoff WL. Ototoxicity of otic drops applied to the middle ear in the chinchilla. Am J Otolaryngol 1984;5:166–76.
99. Wright CG, Halama AR, Meyerhoff WL. Ototoxicity of an ototopical preparation in a primate. Am J Otol 1987;8:56–60.
100. Daniel SJ, Munguia R. Ototoxicity of topical ciprofloxacin/dexamethasone otic suspension in a chinchilla animal model. Otolaryngol Head Neck Surg 2008; 139:840–5.
101. Roland PS, Kreisler LS, Reese B, et al. Topical ciprofloxacin/dexamethasone otic suspension is superior to ofloxacin otic solution in the treatment of children with acute otitis media with otorrhea through tympanostomy tubes. Pediatrics 2004; 113:e40–6.
102. Emgard P, Hellstrom S, Holm S. External otitis caused by infection with *Pseudomonas aeruginosa* or *Candida albicans* cured by use of a topical group III steroid, without any antibiotics. Acta Otolaryngol 2005;125:346–52.
103. Emgard P, Hellstrom S. A topical steroid without an antibiotic cures external otitis efficiently: a study in an animal model. Eur Arch Otorhinolaryngol 2001;258:287–91.
104. Smeraldi R. Clinica e diagnosi di alcune mastoiditi atipichi. Gazz Sanit 1947;18: 58–61.
105. Groth A, Enoksson F, Hultcrantz M, et al. Acute mastoiditis in children aged 0-16 years: a national study of 678 cases in Sweden comparing different age groups. Int J Pediatr Otorhinolaryngol 2012;76(10):1494–500.
106. Holt GR, Gates GA. Masked mastoiditis. Laryngoscope 1983;93:1034–7.
107. Hutchinson CA. Chemotherapy in acute middle-ear disease: "masked mastoiditis". Br Med J 1941;2:159–60.
108. Beers SL, Abramo TJ. Otitis externa review. Pediatr Emerg Care 2004;20:250–6.
109. van den Aardweg MT, Rovers MM, de Ru JA, et al. A systematic review of diagnostic criteria for acute mastoiditis in children. Otol Neurotol 2008;29:751–7.
110. Schwartz RH, Pitkaranta A, Winther B. Computed tomography imaging of the maxillary and ethmoid sinuses in children with short-duration purulent rhinorrhea. Otolaryngol Head Neck Surg 2001;124:160–3.
111. Gwaltney JM Jr, Phillips CD, Miller RD, et al. Computed tomographic study of the common cold. N Engl J Med 1994;330:25–30.
112. Kaiser L, Lew D, Hirschel B, et al. Effects of antibiotic treatment in the subset of common-cold patients who have bacteria in nasopharyngeal secretions. Lancet 1996;347:1507–10.
113. Dhooge IJ, Vandenbussche T, Lemmerling M. Value of computed tomography of the temporal bone in acute otomastoiditis. Rev Laryngol Otol Rhinol (Bord) 1998;119:91–4.
114. Antonelli PJ, Garside JA, Mancuso AA, et al. Computed tomography and the diagnosis of coalescent mastoiditis. Otolaryngol Head Neck Surg 1999;120:350–4.
115. Vazquez E, Castellote A, Piqueras J, et al. Imaging of complications of acute mastoiditis in children. Radiographics 2003;23:359–72. Available at: http://intl-radiographics.rsna.org/content/23/2/359.full.
116. Nadal D, Herrmann P, Baumann A, et al. Acute mastoiditis: clinical, microbiological, and therapeutic aspects. Eur J Pediatr 1990;149:560–4.
117. Gradenigo G. Über die Paralyse des Nervus abducens bei Otitis. Archiv für Ohrenheilkunde 1907;74:149–87.
118. Chole RA, Donald PJ. Petrous apicitis. Clinical considerations. Ann Otol Rhinol Laryngol 1983;92:544–51.
119. Marianowski R, Rocton S, Ait-Amer JL, et al. Conservative management of Gradenigo syndrome in a child. Int J Pediatr Otorhinolaryngol 2001;57:79–83.

120. Rossor TE, Anderson YC, Steventon NB, et al. Conservative management of Gradenigo's syndrome in a child. BMJ Case Rep 2011;2011.
121. Ulkumen B, Kaplan Y. Conservative treatment of Gradenigo's syndrome triggered by acute otitis media. Pak J Med Sci Q 2012;28:735–7.
122. Gaio E, Marioni G, de Filippis C, et al. Facial nerve paralysis secondary to acute otitis media in infants and children. J Paediatr Child Health 2004;40:483–6.
123. Redaelli de Zinis LO, Gamba P, Balzanelli C. Acute otitis media and facial nerve paralysis in adults. Otol Neurotol 2003;24:113–7.
124. Joseph EM, Sperling NM. Facial nerve paralysis in acute otitis media: cause and management revisited. Otolaryngol Head Neck Surg 1998;118:694–6.
125. Roberts DB. The etiology of bullous myringitis and the role of mycoplasmas in ear disease: a review. Pediatrics 1980;65:761–6.
126. McCormick DP, Saeed KA, Pittman C, et al. Bullous myringitis: a case-control study. Pediatrics 2003;112:982–6.
127. Lou ZC, Lou ZH, Zhang QP. Traumatic tympanic membrane perforations: a study of etiology and factors affecting outcome. Am J Otolaryngol 2012;33:549–55.
128. Griffin WL Jr. A retrospective study of traumatic tympanic membrane perforations in a clinical practice. Laryngoscope 1979;89:261–82.
129. Kristensen S. Spontaneous healing of traumatic tympanic membrane perforations in man: a century of experience. J Laryngol Otol 1992;106:1037–50.
130. Ritenour AE, Wickley A, Ritenour JS, et al. Tympanic membrane perforation and hearing loss from blast overpressure in Operation Enduring Freedom and Operation Iraqi Freedom wounded. J Trauma 2008;64:S174–8 [discussion: S8].
131. Pahor AL. The ENT problems following the Birmingham bombings. J Laryngol Otol 1981;95:399–406.
132. Orji FT, Agu CC. Determinants of spontaneous healing in traumatic perforations of the tympanic membrane. Clin Otolaryngol 2008;33:420–6.
133. Ireland PE. Traumatic perforations of tympanic membrane due to blast injury. Can Med Assoc J 1946;54:256–8.
134. Amadasun JE. An observational study of the management of traumatic tympanic membrane perforations. J Laryngol Otol 2002;116:181–4.
135. Roland PS, Stroman DW. Microbiology of acute otitis externa. Laryngoscope 2002;112:1166–77.
136. Martinez Devesa P, Willis CM, Capper JW. External auditory canal pH in chronic otitis externa. Clin Otolaryngol Allied Sci 2003;28:320–4.
137. Stone M, Fulghum RS. Bactericidal activity of wet cerumen. Ann Otol Rhinol Laryngol 1984;93:183–6.
138. Pata YS, Ozturk C, Akbas Y, et al. Has cerumen a protective role in recurrent external otitis? Am J Otolaryngol 2003;24:209–12.
139. Nussinovitch M, Rimon A, Volovitz B, et al. Cotton-tip applicators as a leading cause of otitis externa. Int J Pediatr Otorhinolaryngol 2004;68:433–5.
140. Carfrae MJ, Kesser BW. Malignant otitis externa. Otolaryngol Clin North Am 2008;41:537–49, viii–ix.
141. Ruben RJ. Efficacy of ofloxacin and other otic preparations for otitis externa. Pediatr Infect Dis J 2001;20:108–10 [discussion: 20–2].
142. Osguthorpe JD, Nielsen DR. Otitis externa: review and clinical update. Am Fam Physician 2006;74:1510–6.
143. Myer CM III. The evolution of ototopical therapy: from cumin to quinolones. Ear Nose Throat J 2004;83:9–11.
144. Myer CM III. Historical perspective on the use of otic antimicrobial agents. Pediatr Infect Dis J 2001;20:98–101 [discussion: 20–2].

145. Tsikoudas A, Jasser P, England RJ. Are topical antibiotics necessary in the management of otitis externa? Clin Otolaryngol Allied Sci 2002;27:260–2.
146. Rutka J. Acute otitis externa: treatment perspectives. Ear Nose Throat J 2004; 83:20–1 [discussion: 1–2].
147. Johnston CS, Gaas CA. Vinegar: medicinal uses and antiglycemic effect. MedGenMed 2006;8:61.
148. Eng CY, El-Hawrani AS. The pH of commonly used topical ear drops in the treatment of otitis externa. Ear Nose Throat J 2011;90:160–2.
149. Dohar JE. Evolution of management approaches for otitis externa. Pediatr Infect Dis J 2003;22:299–305 [quiz: 6–8].
150. Thorp MA, Kruger J, Oliver S, et al. The antibacterial activity of acetic acid and Burow's solution as topical otological preparations. J Laryngol Otol 1998;112: 925–8.
151. Kashiwamura M, Chida E, Matsumura M, et al. The efficacy of Burow's solution as an ear preparation for the treatment of chronic ear infections. Otol Neurotol 2004;25:9–13.
152. Hannley MT, Denneny JC III, Holzer SS. Use of ototopical antibiotics in treating 3 common ear diseases. Otolaryngol Head Neck Surg 2000;122:934–40.
153. Rosenfeld RM, Singer M, Wasserman JM, et al. Systematic review of topical antimicrobial therapy for acute otitis externa. Otolaryngol Head Neck Surg 2006; 134:S24–48.
154. Epstein E. Allergy to dermatologic agents. JAMA 1966;198:517–20.
155. Gette MT, Marks JG Jr, Maloney ME. Frequency of postoperative allergic contact dermatitis to topical antibiotics. Arch Dermatol 1992;128:365–7.
156. Dickel H, Taylor JS, Evey P, et al. Delayed readings of a standard screening patch test tray: frequency of "lost," "found," and "persistent" reactions. Am J Contact Dermatitis 2000;11:213–7.
157. Gates GA. Safety of ofloxacin otic and other ototopical treatments in animal models and in humans. Pediatr Infect Dis J 2001;20:104–7 [discussion: 20–2].
158. Wall GM, Stroman DW, Roland PS, et al. Ciprofloxacin 0.3%/dexamethasone 0.1% sterile otic suspension for the topical treatment of ear infections: a review of the literature. Pediatr Infect Dis J 2009;28:141–4.
159. Dohar JE, Garner ET, Nielsen RW, et al. Topical ofloxacin treatment of otorrhea in children with tympanostomy tubes. Arch Otolaryngol Head Neck Surg 1999; 125:537–45.
160. Jones RN, Milazzo J, Seidlin M. Ofloxacin otic solution for treatment of otitis externa in children and adults. Arch Otolaryngol Head Neck Surg 1997;123: 1193–200.
161. Drehobl M, Guerrero JL, Lacarte PR, et al. Comparison of efficacy and safety of ciprofloxacin otic solution 0.2% versus polymyxin B-neomycin-hydrocortisone in the treatment of acute diffuse otitis externa. Curr Med Res Opin 2008;24: 3531–42.
162. Rahman A, Rizwan S, Waycaster C, et al. Pooled analysis of two clinical trials comparing the clinical outcomes of topical ciprofloxacin/dexamethasone otic suspension and polymyxin B/neomycin/hydrocortisone otic suspension for the treatment of acute otitis externa in adults and children. Clin Ther 2007;29: 1950–6.
163. Pistorius B, Westberry K, Drehobl M. Prospective, randomized, comparative trial of ciprofloxacin otic drops, with or without hydrocortisone, vs. polymyxin B-neomycin-hydrocortisone otic suspension in the treatment of otitis externa. Infect Dis Clin Pract 1999;8:387–95.

164. Mraovic M, Canic-Radojlovic M. The activity of ofloxacin against methicillin-resistant *Staphylococcus aureus*. Infection 1986;14(Suppl 4):S231–2.
165. Peterson LR, Cooper I, Willard KE, et al. Activity of twenty-one antimicrobial agents including l-ofloxacin against quinolone-sensitive and -resistant, and methicillin-sensitive and -resistant *Staphylococcus aureus*. Chemotherapy 1994;40:21–5.
166. Kang SL, Rybak MJ, McGrath BJ, et al. Pharmacodynamics of levofloxacin, ofloxacin, and ciprofloxacin, alone and in combination with rifampin, against methicillin-susceptible and -resistant *Staphylococcus aureus* in an in vitro infection model. Antimicrobial Agents Chemother 1994;38:2702–9.
167. Torum B, Block SL, Avila H, et al. Efficacy of ofloxacin otic solution once daily for 7 days in the treatment of otitis externa: a multicenter, open-label, phase III trial. Clin Ther 2004;26:1046–54.
168. Chandler JR. Malignant external otitis. Laryngoscope 1968;78:1257–94.
169. Hern JD, Almeyda J, Thomas DM, et al. Malignant otitis externa in HIV and AIDS. J Laryngol Otol 1996;110:770–5.
170. Gordon G, Giddings NA. Invasive otitis externa due to *Aspergillus* species: case report and review. Clin Infect Dis 1994;19:866–70.
171. Cruveilhier J. Anatomie Pathologique du Corps Humain, Vol. 1, Book 2, Plate 6. Paris: Bailliere; 1829.
172. Harker LA, Koontz FP. Bacteriology of cholesteatoma: clinical significance. Trans Sect Otolaryngol Am Acad Ophthalmol Otolaryngol 1977;84:ORL-683–6.
173. Holt JJ. Ear canal cholesteatoma. Laryngoscope 1992;102:608–13.
174. Hanif J, Frosh A, Marnane C, et al. Lesson of the week: "high" ear piercing and the rising incidence of perichondritis of the pinna. BMJ 2001;322:906–7.
175. Roland PS, Smith TL, Schwartz SR, et al. Clinical practice guideline: cerumen impaction. Otolaryngol Head Neck Surg 2008;139:S1–21.
176. Bressler K, Shelton C. Ear foreign-body removal: a review of 98 consecutive cases. Laryngoscope 1993;103:367–70.
177. Balbani AP, Sanchez TG, Butugan O, et al. Ear and nose foreign body removal in children. Int J Pediatr Otorhinolaryngol 1998;46:37–42.
178. Mackle T, Conlon B. Foreign bodies of the nose and ears in children. Should these be managed in the accident and emergency setting? Int J Pediatr Otorhinolaryngol 2006;70:425–8.
179. DiMuzio J Jr, Deschler DG. Emergency department management of foreign bodies of the external ear canal in children. Otol Neurotol 2002;23:473–5.
180. Davies PH, Benger JR. Foreign bodies in the nose and ear: a review of techniques for removal in the emergency department. J Accid Emerg Med 2000;17:91–4.
181. Hanson RM, Stephens M. Cyanoacrylate-assisted foreign body removal from the ear and nose in children. J Paediatr Child Health 1994;30:77–8.
182. Raz S, Stassen R, Hilding D. Impression materials for removal of aural foreign bodies. Ann Otol Rhinol Laryngol 1977;86:396–9.
183. Wavde V. Removal of foreign body from nose or ear. Aust Fam Physician 1988; 17:904.
184. Stool SE, McConnel CS Jr. Foreign bodies in pediatric otolaryngology. Some diagnostic and therapeutic pointers. Clin Pediatr (Phila) 1973;12:113–6.
185. Brunskill AJ, Satterthwaite K. Foreign bodies. Ann Emerg Med 1994;24:757.
186. Ernst E. Ear candles: a triumph of ignorance over science. J Laryngol Otol 2004; 118:1–2.
187. Seely DR, Quigley SM, Langman AW. Ear candles: efficacy and safety. Laryngoscope 1996;106:1226–9.

Epistaxis: An Overview

Zachary A. Kasperek, MD[a],*, Gary F. Pollock, MD[a,b]

KEYWORDS

- Epistaxis • Anterior packing • Posterior packing • Nosebleed

KEY POINTS

- History and physical examination should be able to locate the source of bleeding. One should then tailor further management accordingly.
- Most bleeds are anterior, and most anterior bleeds are amenable to cautery.
- Be aware of the risk of hypotension and hypoxia with any posterior packing, and treat these patients with caution.
- If tamponade is required, commercially available balloon tamponade devices are quickly deployed, well tolerated, and easy to remove.

Although epistaxis is rarely a cause of mortality,[1] it leads to morbidity in select patient groups and represents a frequently encountered otolaryngologic emergency.[2]

ANATOMY

Epistaxis is classified as either anterior or posterior. Anterior epistaxis is defined as bleeding from the anterior nasal septum, an area known as the Kiesselbach plexus. This area has branches of the superior labial artery, sphenopalatine artery, anterior ethmoid artery, and posterior ethmoid artery, along with the greater palatine artery. The area is supplied by end branches of both the internal and external carotid arteries, with the internal supplying the ethmoids and the external supplying the sphenopalatine and palatine along with the superior labial via the facial artery.[3] Posterior epistaxis typically arises from the sphenopalatine artery, which flows from the external carotid; however, it may also originate in the descending palatine arteries[4] or the internal carotid artery itself.[5] These bleeds typically occur along the nasal septum or lateral nasal wall.

Funding Sources: None.
Conflict of Interest: None.
[a] Emergency Medicine Residency, University of Pittsburgh, 230 McKee Place, Suite 500, Pittsburgh, PA 15213, USA; [b] UPMC Mercy Hospital, 1400 Locust Street, Pittsburgh, PA 15219, USA
* Corresponding author.
E-mail address: kasperekza@upmc.edu

Emerg Med Clin N Am 31 (2013) 443–454
http://dx.doi.org/10.1016/j.emc.2013.01.008
0733-8627/13/$ – see front matter © 2013 Elsevier Inc. All rights reserved.

emed.theclinics.com

INCIDENCE

Epistaxis has been reported to cause 1.7 emergency department (ED) visits per 100,000 population.[6] It has a bimodal age distribution, with peaks at younger than 10 and between 70 and 79 years of age. With the largest percentage of ED visits due to epistaxis occurring in those age 70 to 79 years, this will become a more frequent cause of emergency visits as the population ages. Posterior nosebleeds tend to be more common in older patients.[7]

ETIOLOGY

Epistaxis can be caused by a wide variety of factors (**Box 1**). In the younger age groups, digital trauma is the most frequent cause.[8] Mucosal trauma from topical nasal drugs, such as antihistamines and corticosteroids, may result in anterior epistaxis. Dry air from indoor heating during the winter months likely accounts for the peak in incidence during this time period.[9] This dryness also likely accounts for the increased frequency in those wearing intranasal oxygen. Significant epistaxis can also result from nasal or septal trauma and can be associated with underlying nasal bone fractures. Illicit drug insufflation can result in epistaxis caused by local trauma, inflammation, or vasoactive effects from these substances.[10] Several other entities have been implicated in the cause of epistaxis including septal perforations, viral or bacterial rhinosinusitis, and neoplasms. Iatrogenic causes can occur as secondary to nasotracheal intubation, insertion of a gastric tube, or nasal airway or other instrumentation.

In addition to local causes, systemic conditions associated with coagulopathies can also be associated with epistaxis. These conditions can include genetic disorders such as hemophilia, acquired coagulopathies due to renal or liver disease, hematologic cancers, or the use of anticoagulant medications. Low-dose aspirin appears to increase the risk of epistaxis slightly.[11] In one study of patients with epistaxis requiring admission, cardiovascular and idiopathic causes were considered by the treating otolaryngologist to be the most common.[12] There are no known specific conditions or risk factors associated with posterior nose bleeds.[7]

The literature is unclear regarding any association between hypertension and epistaxis, with the possible exception that there may be some correlation between poorly controlled hypertension and epistaxis.[13–16]

MANAGEMENT

Although rarely life-threatening, the initial management of epistaxis should focus on the evaluation and stabilization of the airway, breathing, and circulation of the patient. Ensuring hemodynamic stability and patency of the airway is paramount, and resuscitative efforts should take initial priority over stopping the nosebleed. Universal precautions must be taken in all cases of epistaxis to protect the health care provider from blood-borne illness, and full protection including a facemask and eye protection is recommended. Important points in the history include previous episodes, laterality of the nosebleed, trauma, coagulopathy (physiologic, familial, or pharmacologic), duration, and severity. Warning signs of severe blood loss such as lightheadedness, chest pain, syncope, and shortness of breath should be elicited. On physical examination it is often helpful to have tissues available and have the patient blow the nose to evacuate the clot before the examination. Inspect the nasal mucosa, with the aid of nasal speculum, for the source of the bleeding. If the source is not identified, inspect the posterior oropharynx for signs of blood, as this may point to a posterior cause of epistaxis. It may be helpful to have the patient gargle with water before

Box 1
Causes of epistaxis

- Acquired
- Congenital
  - Septal deviation
  - Septal spur
- Vascular
  - Hereditary hemorrhagic telangiectasia
  - Wegner granulomatosis
  - Hypertension
  - Congestive heart failure
- Inflammatory
  - Rhinosinusitis
  - Nasal polyps
  - Nasal diphtheria
- Trauma/toxin
  - Nose picking
  - Facial trauma
  - Foreign body
  - Illicit insufflations
  - Septal perforation
  - Barotrauma
- Autoimmune
  - Hemophilia
  - Leukemia
  - Von Willebrand disease
- Metabolic
  - Uremia
  - Liver failure
  - Alcohol
- Idiopathic
- Iatrogenic
  - Antiplatelet agents (aspirin, clopidogrel, dipyridamole)
  - Anticoagulant agents (heparin, warfarin)
  - Thrombolytics
  - Nonsteroidal anti-inflammatory drugs
  - Intranasal medications
  - Postsurgical
  - Nasal passage of tubes (nasotracheal intubation, nasogastric drainage)
- Neoplastic
  - Juvenile angiofibroma
  - Squamous cell cancer
  - Paranasal sinus tumor

this step to clear the oropharynx of any dried blood and more clearly identify new blood.

Initial management can begin simultaneously with the physical examination and history. Application of a topical vasoconstrictor with the patient applying bilateral, pinching pressure just caudal to the bridge of the nose is often effective in stopping anterior bleeds, at least temporarily. Application of a topical anesthetic and vasoconstrictor (**Box 2**) may be useful to ensure patient comfort and control the bleeding enough to allow for a thorough physical examination. In patients unable to tolerate examination, cautious use of oral or parenteral anxiolytics and analgesics may be helpful, but generally would be reserved for special circumstances. However, if they are used, one must be prepared to manage and potential complications and effects from these medications.

ANTERIOR EPISTAXIS

Definitive management should proceed once the source is identified. Anterior bleeds are often amenable to cautery, most often accomplished with silver nitrate on applicator sticks. Important points to remember when using this method are that this should only be performed unilaterally, it should only be used for small areas of bleeding, and only a brief application (around 5 seconds or less) should be used.[17] Situations other than these involve an increased risk of perforation. Another important point concerning silver nitrate cautery is that the septum must be dry and free of "wet" blood or clot before application. A good way to achieve this and a modicum of anesthesia is intranasal application of mixture of 1:1 phenylephrine and 4% viscous lidocaine. This agent can be applied to cotton balls or cotton dental roll gauze and then inserted into the affected nares for 10 to 20 minutes to achieve its effects before attempting cautery. After cautery it is useful to apply a topical antibiotic ointment or petroleum jelly to the affected area to keep it moist, with the patient instructed to apply ointment or use nasal saline 3 to 4 times daily to prevent desiccation and rebleeding.

For anterior bleeds that do not seem amenable to cautery or whereby cautery has failed, packing can be useful. There are many ways and many products available to pack a nose, one of the most commonly available being petroleum gauze. Bayonet forceps and a nasal speculum are necessary to perform this procedure. In addition, a well-functioning headlamp is ideal to free the clinician's hands to perform the procedure and allow for adequate visualization. When layering the Vaseline gauze, ensure to do so in an "accordion" fashion. Packing may be performed in a medial to lateral or caudal to

---

Box 2
Commonly used topical medications

Topical Vasoconstrictors

- Phenylephrine (0.5%–1%)
- Cocaine 4%
- Oxymetazoline (Afrin)
- Epinephrine (1:1000)

Topical Anesthetics

- Cocaine 4%
- Lidocaine 4%
- Procaine 2%

cephalad direction. When layering the Vaseline gauze one must make sure to grasp more than twice the length of the nares so as to allow for appropriate folding (**Fig. 1**).

There is also a variety of commercial products available for the packing of anterior bleeds, which all seem to be well tolerated and are more quickly applied, thus making them an attractive option. Medtronic (Minneapolis, MN) makes a variety of nasal tampons made of polyvinyl alcohol, a compressed polymer that is "inflated" with saline administration, under the Merocel moniker. A competing nasal tampon is made by Shippert Medical Technologies Corporation (Centennial, CO) under the Rhino-Rocket moniker. When using these devices it is important to choose the proper size or trim the tampon to the size for the nares, to prevent discomfort, before application. The tampon is then lubricated using antibiotic ointment or non–water-soluble lubricant and inserted into the affected nares in one smooth motion. Bayonet forceps and a nasal speculum may aid with insertion. The tampon is then moistened with saline to inflate. One way to ensure equal inflation is to attach an 18-gauge angio-catheter to a 20-mL syringe, fill with saline, then start moistening in a posterior to anterior fashion using the angio-catheter. Sometimes 2 tampons must be used to fill the entire cavity. In addition, tampons can also be cut in half and used in the same fashion.[18] If an attached suture is present, this may be taped to the ipsilateral cheek to facilitate removal on follow-up. It is important to instruct the patient to keep the nasal tampon moist via the use of saline nasal drops while the packing is in place. Both of these types of tampon are constructed of polyvinyl acetate (PVA) and work by expanding and placing direct pressure on the source of bleeding, and therefore must be situated over the top of the vessel.

There is also a way of crafting nasal tampons from salt pork, which has been shown to be effective in the past and has recently been rediscovered.[19,20]

Balloon devices are also available for nasal packing. ArthroCare Corporation (Austin, TX) makes a variety of devices under the Rapid Rhino moniker. These products are high-volume, low-pressure devices, have a self-lubricating hydrocolloid outer coating, contain a pilot balloon for pressure checking, and are recommended to be inflated with air by the manufacturer. The devices are soaked briefly in sterile water and then inserted into the affected nares, usually without any additional equipment necessary. Once inserted, the pilot balloon is inflated to an appropriate pressure. The pilot balloon is then usually taped to the ipsilateral cheek. There are studies showing improved patient comfort with this pack in comparison with the Merocel tampon.[21]

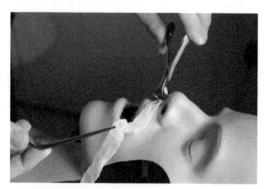

Fig. 1. Demonstration of petroleum gauze packing technique, including grasping twice the length of the nare for packing and correct positioning of the nasal speculum in a cranial-caudal orientation, as opposed to medial-lateral orientation.

Bilateral packing may sometimes be required to achieve adequate pressure for bleeding that is difficult to control. By packing bilateral nares one may achieve greater pressure over the source of the bleeding. If bilateral packing is required admission should be considered, as this has been shown to decrease oxygen saturation and increase heart rate in healthy patients.[22] Those with significant comorbidities may therefore be placed at risk by this procedure and should be adequately monitored during and after the procedure.

For anterior bleeds whereby cautery and packing have failed or are impractical for whatever reason, there is a variety of products for cessation of bleeding. There is an isolated case report of QuikClot,[23] a kaolin-impregnated rayon/polyester gauze, used for this purpose. Kaolin activates Factor XII, thus activating the intrinsic clotting pathway and encouraging a local clot to form over the source of bleeding. In this case report the gauze was left in place for 1 week before removal, with good results and no rebleeding. When leaving any packing in place in the nose it is important to instruct the patient to keep the pack moist, and this case is no exception. It is worth noting that QuikClot is currently approved by the Food and Drug Administration traumatic external hemorrhage only.

HemCon Medical Technologies produces both a bandage and a gelfoam using chitosan, a polysaccharide derived from shrimp. This process seems to work via covalent interactions as the chitosan exposes a positively charged matrix to which negatively charged surfaces of red blood cells are then attracted, leading to the creation of a plug that can arrest bleeding. There have been trials using this bandage wrapped around a typical PVA tampon for treatment failures,[24] and using the gel foam directly applied to bleeding areas in sheep,[25] which show promise.

Baxter (Hayward, CA) produces a product made of thrombin impregnated into gelatin granules, known as Floseal. It works via the topical effect of the thrombin cleaving fibrinogen in the patients' blood to fibrin and also through a pressure effect produced as the gelatin granules swell when hydrated. It has been shown in manufacturer-supported research to be more convenient, better tolerated, and subjectively more effective than packing.[26]

POSTERIOR EPISTAXIS

If anterior packing fails to resolve the bleeding, or ongoing bleeding is noted in the posterior oropharynx after anterior packing, a posterior source must be considered. As for anterior nosebleeds, several methods to pack a posterior source have been described.

The classic method for packing a posterior source involves red rubber catheters, silk suture, long forceps, rolls of gauze, and a method of anterior packing. Bilateral nasopharynx and the posterior oropharynx are anesthetized with aerosolized and/or topical anesthetic. A roll of gauze is introduced via the oropharynx and secured in the posterior oropharynx using the silk sutures and red rubber catheters. One or both anterior nasal cavities can then be packed in whichever fashion is preferred, as needed, to control bleeding and stabilize the nasopharynx.[27]

Another method of tamponading the posterior nasopharynx using commonly available equipment uses a Foley catheter. The Foley catheter is advanced into the posterior oropharynx and partially inflated, then pulled anteriorly to create pressure posteriorly. If there is significant pain or deviation of the soft palate with inflation, one must stop immediately and reassess to ensure that the catheter is in the proper location (**Fig. 2**). It is usually necessary to then pack the affected anterior nares. The Foley catheter can then be clamped in place using an umbilical clamp

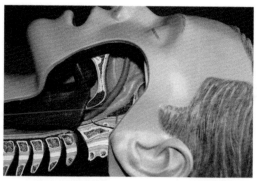

Fig. 2. Demonstration of Foley catheter tamponade technique. Notice the tip of the catheter in the posterior oropharynx. At this point the catheter may be inflated and the opposite end withdrawn from the nare to tamponade posterior bleeding.

or nasogastric tube clamp, with gauze to serve as padding over the soft tissues of the nose.

There are also commercially available products for dealing with posterior epistaxis. These products typically have two ports, one for an anterior balloon and one for a posterior balloon. The devices are inserted, the posterior balloon inflated and snugged forward to tamponade the bleeding, then the anterior balloon is inflated to maintain placement.

Medtronic makes a product line known as Epistat and ArthroCare makes one known as Rhino Rocket. The Epistat I and Rhino Rocket are very similar, save for the lack of coating material on the Epistat, which therefore can be lubricated with sterile lubricant, water, or saline, unlike the Rhino Rocket, which should be soaked in sterile water. In general, it is recommended to pack the contralateral nares to prevent septal deviation; however, the evidence to back up this recommendation is lacking. The Epistat II is a posterior balloon with an anterior Merocel tampon, both of which are operated as mentioned previously.

COMPLICATIONS

A potential complication of both cauterization and packing is septal perforation, caused by direct effects in the former and pressure necrosis in the later. Other potential complications of any interventions include patient discomfort, which can be managed on an outpatient basis with oral acetaminophen and/or opiates. In some cases, patient discomfort may be refractory to these interventions and may require admission for intravenous analgesia or anxiolytics.

Any form of packing can create a walled-off cavity in the sinuses, thus predisposing to infection. This situation creates the potential risk of toxic shock syndrome[28] or sinusitis, therefore it has been customarily recommended to place all patients with nasal packing on antibiotics to prevent these complications.[29] Amoxicillin, cephalexin, or amoxicillin-clavulanate should be sufficient, depending on local resistance patterns. Clindamycin can be used for penicillin-allergic patients. If signs and symptoms of toxic shock syndrome do appear (nausea, vomiting, hypotension, elevated temperature, erythroderma), it is important to discontinue the packing immediately and continue antibiotics directed toward a presumed *Staphylococcus aureus* infection.

Posterior packing can increase vagal tone, leading to bradycardia and hypotension, and can also lead to hypoventilation[30] or aspiration from dislodgment or malpositioning.[31] Therefore it has customarily been recommended to admit all patients with posterior nasal packing for monitoring and analgesia.

GENERAL NOTES

For patients with platelet dysfunction, or inherited or acquired bleeding disorders, it may be helpful to use appropriate blood products (fresh frozen plasma, platelets) or recombinant Factor VIIa (NovoSeven), although data for such practice is lacking. Recombinant Factor VIIa has been shown to be effective in slowing nasal bleeding in these populations.[32,33] The evidence cannot currently recommend its use outside of these selected patient groups.[34] Given the potential significant side effects and risks of these interventions and products, a risk/benefit analysis must be assessed in each patient by the clinician considering using those products. A transfusion of packed red blood cells must be considered in those patients with significant bleeding, anemia, or ongoing blood loss.

For many patients, local vasoconstriction and analgesia is all that is necessary to facilitate packing. However, some patients are unable to tolerate packing placement without further analgesia. The otolaryngology literature recommends nonsteroidal anti-inflammatory drugs (NSAIDs) before removal of nasal packings.[35,36] Acetaminophen, NSAIDs, and opiates can all be considered for pain control in these patients. There is a risk of potential platelet inhibition with NSAID use, which should be considered in anyone with ongoing bleeding. Alternatively, opiates can have a sedative effect and can lead to other side effects such as nausea and emesis, so the clinician may need to have an informed discussion with the patient weighing the risks and benefits of the various options for analgesia. As with any painful procedure, sedation and analgesia may also be necessary to facilitate packing; however, one must be prepared to deal with the side effects and potential complications of these medications, including potential respiratory compromise. Finally, it is occasionally impossible to place posterior packing without full sedation, and general anesthesia and endotracheal intubation are sometimes required.

All packing should be left in place for 3 to 5 days. If available, it is helpful to refer the patient to an otolaryngology specialist for packing removal in case the packing proves unsuccessful and further measures are necessary to control the bleed. However, many primary care providers are comfortable managing these patients in their offices, and a call to ensure adequate follow-up can be helpful.

Regarding hypertension, there is no consensus in the literature regarding the necessity of treatment for the control of epistaxis. If the patient is having difficulty controlling epistaxis and is also hypertensive, it may be prudent to attempt lowering the blood pressure while additional attempts at hemostasis are being undertaken.[37] Anxiolysis and analgesia may also assist in managing the patient's elevated blood pressure if it is secondary to pain and patient discomfort within the situation and treatment.

For epistaxis not amenable to packing there are alternatives, including surgical ligation of vessels,[38] angiographic embolization of vessels,[39] hot-water irrigation,[40] septal surgery, endoscopic electrocautery,[41] fibrin glue,[42] and laser treatment[43]; however these procedures should only be attempted in concert with an otolaryngology specialist, and are therefore outside the purview of this article. Surgical and angiographic measures have never been shown to have benefits as regards improved costs, risk/benefit, morbidity, or mortality when compared with packing,[44,45] therefore packing should be attempted first; however, some bleeds are not amenable to packing and will require further advanced measures.

Box 3
Helpful equipment for the evaluation of epistaxis

- Reclinable chair with headrest
- Headlamp
- Tissues
- Kidney basin
- Nasal speculum
- Yankauer and Frazier suction tips
- Gown, gloves, face mask

RECOMMENDED APPROACH

As there are no large, placebo-controlled, randomized trials of epistaxis treatment, the authors are only able to recommend an approach that is a matter of expert opinion (level B). **Boxes 3** and **4** list the recommended equipment to have available.

The authors' recommended approach includes history and physical examination as outlined earlier, followed by intranasal application of topical lidocaine and phenylephrine, which their pharmacy provides for the ED in prefilled syringes, followed by silver nitrate cautery (if it is not a large area of bleeding). If this is unsuccessful, use of an anterior nasal packing balloon system is well tolerated, quick, and usually effective. If this is unsuccessful, either bilateral anterior packing or a balloon posterior packing system is recommended, depending on the presumed source. Once first-line packing has failed it is often helpful to obtain telephone consultation with the otolaryngology specialist on call, as these patients are more likely to require further measures to control their bleeding and thus will require close follow-up.

Box 4
Helpful equipment for the management of epistaxis

Anterior:

- Silver nitrate sticks
- Antibiotic ointment
- Dental rolls or cotton balls
- Topical vasoconstrictors/anesthetics
- Bayonet forceps
- Vaseline gauze (0.5 × 72 in; 1.3 × 183 cm)
- Prepackaged nasal balloons/tampons
- Surgicel/Gelfoam

Posterior:

- 2 Foley catheters
- Gauze
- 3 silk sutures
- Umbilical clamp
- Prepackaged anterior/posterior packing system

REFERENCES

1. Woolf C, Jacobs A. Epistaxis mortality. J Laryngol Otol 1961;75:114–22.
2. Bleach N, Williamson P, Mady S. Emergency workload in otolaryngology. Ann R Coll Surg Engl 1994;76:335–8.
3. Koh E, Frazzini V, Kagetsu N. Epistaxis: vascular anatomy, origins, and endovascular treatment. AJR Am J Roentgenol 2000;174:845–51.
4. Viehweg T, Roberson J, Hudson J. Epistaxis: diagnosis and treatment. J Oral Maxillofac Surg 2006;64:511–8.
5. Teitelbaum G, Halbach V, Larsen D, et al. Treatment of massive posterior epistaxis by detachable coil embolization of a cavernous internal carotid artery aneurysm. Neuroradiology 1995;37:334–6.
6. Pallin D, Chng Y, McKay M, et al. Epidemiology of epistaxis in US emergency departments, 1992 to 2001. Ann Emerg Med 2005;46:77–81.
7. Viducich R, Blanda M, Gerson L. Posterior epistaxis: clinical features and acute complications. Ann Emerg Med 1995;25(5):592–6.
8. Gilyoma J, Chalya P. Etiological profile and treatment outcome of epistaxis at a tertiary care hospital in Northwestern Tanzania: a prospective review of 104 cases. BMC Ear Nose Throat Disord 2011;11:8.
9. Walker T, Macfarlane T, McGarry G. The epidemiology and chronobiology of epistaxis: an investigation of Scottish hospital admission 1995-2004. Clin Otolaryngol 2007;32:361–5.
10. Jewers W, Rawal Y, Allen C. Palatal perforation associated with intranasal prescription narcotic abuse. Oral Surg Oral Med Oral Pathol Oral Radiol Endod 2005;99:594–7.
11. Ridker PM, Cook NR, Lee IM, et al. A randomized trial of low-dose aspirin in the primary prevention of cardiovascular disease in women. N Engl J Med 2005;352:1293–304.
12. Varshney S, Saxena R. Epistaxis: a retrospective clinical study. Indian J Otolaryngol Head Neck Surg 2005;57(2):125–9.
13. Herkner H, Havel C, Mullner M, et al. Active epistaxis at ED presentation is associated with arterial hypertension. Am J Emerg Med 2000;20:92–5.
14. Herkner H, Laggner A, Mullner M. Hypertension in patients presenting with epistaxis. Ann Emerg Med 2000;35:126–30.
15. Neto J, Fuchs F, Facco S, et al. Is epistaxis evidence of end-organ damage in patients with hypertension. Laryngoscope 1999;109:1111–5.
16. Fuchs F, Moreira L, Pires C, et al. Absence of associate between hypertension and epistaxis: a population-based study. Blood Press 2003;12:145–8.
17. Hanif J, Tasca R, Frosh A. Silver nitrate: histological effects of cautery on epithelial surfaces with varying contact times. Clin Otolaryngol Allied Sci 2003;28:368–70.
18. Visvanathan V. Anterior nasal packing with Merocel: a modification. Clin Otolaryngol 2008;33:510.
19. Humphreys I, Saraiya S, Belenky W. Nasal packing with strips of cured pork as treatment for uncontrollable epistaxis in a patient with Glanzmann thrombasthenia. Ann Otol Rhinol Laryngol 2011;120:732–6.
20. Cone A. Use of salt pork in cases of hemorrhage. Arch Otolaryngol Head Neck Surg 1940;32(5):941–6.
21. Moulmoulidis I, Draper M, Patel H. A prospective randomised controlled trial comparing Merocel and Rapid Rhino nasal tampons in the treatment of epistaxis. Eur Arch Otorhinolaryngol 2006;263(8):719–22.

22. Ögretmenoglu O, Yılmaz T, Rahimi K. The effect on arterial blood gases and heart rate of bilateral nasal packing. Eur Arch Otorhinolaryngol 2002;259(2):63–6.

23. Gurdeep S, Harvinder S, Amanjit K. Intranasal use of Quikclot in a patient with uncontrollable epistaxis. Med J Malaysia 2006;61(1):112–3.

24. Shikani A, Chahine K, Alqudah M. Endoscopically guided chitosan nasal packing for intractable epistaxis. Am J Rhinol Allergy 2011;25(1):61–3.

25. Valentine R, Athanasiadis T, Moratti S. The efficacy of a novel chitosan gel on hemostasis after endoscopic sinus surgery in a sheep model of chronic rhinosinusitis. Am J Rhinol Allergy 2009;23:71–5.

26. Mathiasen R, Cruz R. Prospective, randomized, controlled, clinical trial of a novel matrix hemostatic sealant in patients with acute anterior epistaxis. Laryngoscope 2005;115(5):899–902.

27. Riviello R, Brown A. Otolaryngologic procedures. In: Roberts J, Hedges J, editors. Clinical procedures in emergency medicine. 5th edition. Philadelphia: Saunders Elsevier; 2010. p. 1204–7.

28. Jacobson J, Kasworm E. Toxic shock syndrome after nasal surgery. Arch Otolaryngol Head Neck Surg 1986;112:329–32.

29. Hull H, Mann J, Sands J. Toxic shock syndrome related to nasal packing. Arch Otolaryngol 1983;109(9):624–6.

30. Cassisi N, Biller H, Joseph O. Changes in arterial oxygen tension and pulmonary mechanics with the use of posterior packing in epistaxis: a preliminary report. Laryngoscope 1971;81(8):1261–6.

31. Williams M, Onslow J. Airway difficulties associated with severe epistaxis. Anaesthesia 1999;54:812–3.

32. Peters M, Heijboer H. Treatment of a patient with Bernard-Soulier syndrome and recurrent nosebleeds with recombinant factor VIIa. Thromb Haemost 1998;80(2): 352.

33. Tengborn L, Petruson B. A patient with Glanzmann thrombasthenia and epistaxis successfully treated with recombinant factor VIIa. Thromb Haemost 1996;75(6): 981–2.

34. Levi M, Peters M, Buller H. Efficacy and safety of recombinant factor VIIa for treatment of severe bleeding: a systematic review. Crit Care Med 2005;33:883–90.

35. Laing M, Clark L. Analgesia and removal of nasal packing. Clin Otolaryngol Allied Sci 1990;15(4):339–42.

36. Yilmazer C, Sener M, Yilmaz I, et al. Pre-emptive analgesia for removal of nasal packing: a double-blind placebo controlled study. Auris Nasus Larynx 2007; 34(4):471–5.

37. Jackson K, Jackson R. Factors associated with active, refractory epistaxis. Arch Otolaryngol Head Neck Surg 1988;114:862–5.

38. Snyderman C, Goldman S, Carrau R, et al. Endoscopic sphenopalatine artery ligation is an effective method of treatment for posterior epistaxis. Am J Rhinol 1999;13(2):137–40.

39. Elahi M, Parnes L, Fox A, et al. Therapeutic embolization the treatment of intractable epistaxis. Arch Otolaryngol Head Neck Surg 1995;121:65–9.

40. Stangerup S, Dommerby H, Siim C, et al. New modification of hot-water irrigation in the treatment of posterior epistaxis. Arch Otolaryngol Head Neck Surg 1999; 125:686–90.

41. Elwany S, Abdel-Fatah H. Endoscopic control of posterior epistaxis. J Laryngol Otol 1996;110:432–4.

42. Vaiman M, Segal S, Eviatar E. Fibrin glue treatment for epistaxis. Rhinology 2002; 40(2):88–91.

43. Siegel M, Keane W, Atkins J, et al. Control of epistaxis in patients with hereditary hemorrhagic telangiectasia. Otolaryngol Head Neck Surg 1991;105(5):675–9.
44. Barlow D, Deleyiannis F, Pinczower E. Effectiveness of surgical management of epistaxis at a tertiary care center. Laryngoscope 1997;107:21–4.
45. Schaitkin B, Strauss M, Houck J. Epistaxis: medical versus surgical therapy: a comparison of efficacy, complication, and economic considerations. Laryngoscope 1987;97:1392–6.

Evaluation and Management of Oral Lesions in the Emergency Department

Alisa M. Gibson, MD, DMD*, Sarah K. Sommerkamp, MD, RDMS

KEYWORDS

- Oral lesion • Herpes simplex virus • Coxsackie virus • Bullous pemphigoid
- Pemphigus vulgaris • Behçet disease • Aphthous ulcers • Tori

KEY POINTS

- A good history and physical examination include full examination of the oral cavity.
- Oral lesions can be categorized into red, white, and black lesions.
- An oral lesion may be the first symptom of a systemic disease (eg, measles, ulcerative colitis, acute leukemia).
- The amount of pain is not commensurate with the deadliness of the condition (aphthous ulcers are painful but benign; malignancy is painless and deadly).
- Herpes simplex virus does not cause aphthous ulcers.
- Oral erosions may signify significant disease such as pemphigus or Stevens-Johnson syndrome/toxic epidural necrolysis.
- Differentiating between many different kinds of lesions, and thereby excluding malignancy, requires biopsy.
- Be suspicious of persistent lesions, because they may be cancer; refer the patient for biopsy.
- Follow-up is essential for all oral lesions.

THE NATURE OF THE PROBLEM

Oral lesions are common but are often difficult for emergency physicians to diagnose. The oral cavity is an unfamiliar area to most physicians, but, given the diverse and potentially deadly systemic diseases that can present first in the mouth, accurate assessment and management are imperative. Oral lesions have a wide causal spectrum, from the medically insignificant (such as geographic tongue) to life threatening (such as Steven-Johnson or oral melanoma). Because of this complexity, oral

Department of Emergency Medicine, University of Maryland School of Medicine, 110 South Paca Street, 6th Floor, Suite 200, Baltimore, MD 21201, USA
* Corresponding author.
E-mail address: alisagibson@umem.org

Emerg Med Clin N Am 31 (2013) 455–463
http://dx.doi.org/10.1016/j.emc.2013.02.004
0733-8627/13/$ – see front matter © 2013 Elsevier Inc. All rights reserved.

medicine is a specialty. Many of these conditions are amenable to outpatient referral; however, the emergency physician must be able to identify lesions that require immediate intervention.

PATIENT HISTORY AND EXAMINATION

Given the numerous types of oral lesions, the medical history of patients with oral lesions and the results of physical examinations are varied. However, the emergency physician's approach to patients with oral lesions should be routine and consistent. Important points are highlighted in **Box 1**.

The physical examination can be focused on the head and neck, but it is important to look for clues of systemic involvement as well. Patients with oral complaints often are triaged to urgent care, so a complete set of vital signs might not have been obtained. Much information can be gleaned from the patient's general appearance: a toxic appearance or cachexia should trigger a more in-depth work-up. It is often best to start outside the mouth to avoid missing important physical findings. Skin lesions may be present with infection or autoimmune conditions, but the patient may not be aware of them (or connect them with their oral complaint) unless asked or examined. Genital lesions or ocular findings are both common with autoimmune conditions. Palpate the neck for lymphadenopathy, which may be present with infection, autoimmune disorders, or malignancy.

The oral examination should include the external portion (the lips) and the intraoral portion (the oral cavity). Most oral lesions do not involve the lips. Exceptions include herpes simplex virus (HSV), cheilitis, and carcinoma. For the intraoral examination, it is important to note color. Most oral pathology textbooks classify oral lesions based on color (eg, red, white). Also note whether ulceration is present, the size of any lesions that are present, and the number of lesions (single vs multiple). Few diseases present on keratinized mucosa, so lesions seen there can narrow the differential diagnosis to HSV, Coxsackie virus (hand/foot/mouth disease), and malignancy. A thorough examination of the tongue is crucial and involves an extra step. Using a piece of gauze, grasp the tongue and pull it partially out of the mouth to allow a good view.

Mucosa within the oral cavity is separated into keratinized, specialized, and nonkeratinized tissue. The hard palate and the attached gingiva constitute the keratinized oral

---

Box 1
Information to be gathered from the patient with oral lesions during the history and physical examination

Onset

Duration

Character (painful or not)

Recurrence (many oral lesions are recurrent)

Close contacts with someone with similar symptoms

Systemic symptoms

Presence of genital lesions

Social history (particularly alcohol and tobacco use and risk factors for human immunodeficiency syndrome virus)

Family history (for autoimmune disorders)

mucosa. The taste buds on the dorsum of the tongue are specialized mucosa; nonkeratinized mucosa is everything else in the oral cavity. The external lips are not mucosa; they are covered by squamous epithelium. The complex salivary system has 2 major ducts. The Stensen duct, the major duct of the parotid gland, is located on the buccal mucosa, opposite the second upper molar. The Wharton duct, the major duct of the submandibular gland, is located on the floor of the mouth, near the frenulum of the tongue.

ERYTHEMATOUS LESIONS

Erythematous lesions can be caused by infection, an autoimmune disease or hypersensitivity, or malignancy. They can also be benign masses.

Infection

Oral lesions can indicate infection with HSV, varicella zoster virus (VZV), Coxsackie virus, human immunodeficiency virus (HIV), or *Treponema pallidum*.

Oral herpes simplex infections can be either type 1 or type 2. Type 1 infection is more common in the mouth; type 2 typically affects the genitals. Both types appear as vesicular lesions and erosions bordered by an erythematous base. Primary infection can be severe and often involves the buccal mucosa as well as the lips. It can be accompanied by flulike systemic symptoms. Recurrent infections are almost exclusively confined to keratinized tissue and typically appear in the same location. Prodromal symptoms (pain, burning, tingling) are common. Triggers include trauma, sunlight, and stress. The diagnosis is typically based on the clinical findings. Specific tests are available, for example, Tzanck smear, herpes culture, and HSV-1 and HSV-2 immunoglobulin (Ig) G/IgM serum markers, but they have limited usefulness in the emergency department (ED) setting.

Treatment of primary infection includes antiviral therapy (acyclovir, valacyclovir, or famciclovir) and pain management, such as magic mouthwash and nonsteroidal anti-inflammatory drugs (NSAIDs) (**Table 1**). Particularly in children, parenteral pain medication and hospital admission may be required if the patient is unable to eat. Recurrences should be managed symptomatically unless the patient is presenting with a clear prodrome, in which case antiviral therapy can be considered. Antiviral medications can be helpful if they are started during the phase of viral replication, before lesion development; they have a role in chronic suppressive therapy.[3–5]

VZV presents as grouped vesicles or erosions that can appear on the hard palate, buccal mucosa, tongue, or gingiva. Chicken pox is generally diagnosed based on the characteristic skin rash. The management of oral lesions is the same as for the rash, with the possible addition of local pain management.

Table 1 Medications for oral lesions	
Name	**Instructions**
Magic mouthwash: diphenhydramine, 12.5 mg/5 mL, mixed with magnesia-alumina and viscous lidocaine in a 1:1:1 ratio[1]	5–10 mL, swish and spit every 2 h as needed for pain
Triamcinolone acetonide, 0.1%, in benzocaine paste, 20%[2]	Apply to ulcer 2 to 4 times daily until healed
Fluocinonide gel, 0.05%[2]	Apply to ulcer 2 to 4 times daily until healed
Amlexanox, 5%, oral paste[2]	Apply to ulcer 2 to 4 times daily until healed

Coxsackie virus (also known as hand, foot, and mouth disease) presents as intraoral and palmar/plantar lesions. Small aphthae tend to be located on the hard and soft palate. Involvement of the lips is rare, and a clear distinction from HSV. Diagnosis is primarily based on the clinical findings, specifically on the location of the lesions and the presence of viral symptoms. Treatment is supportive.

HIV infection is associated with a great many oral disorders, including several erythematous lesions. Patients with primary HIV infection may have painful mucocutaneous ulcers. Oral lesions can also be caused by opportunistic infections (including mucormycosis, cytomegalovirus [CMV], aspergillosis, and leishmaniasis). Kaposi sarcoma involves the oral cavity in 30% of patients.[6] Differentiation of oral ulcers from CMV infection, primary HIV infection, and other infections, as well as malignancy, depends on appropriate referral and biopsy. Management of most of these conditions is contingent on improving patients' autoimmune function and must be done in conjunction with infectious disease specialists.

Syphilis may present as a characteristic chancre that is commonly thought of as presenting on the genitals but can occur in the mouth as well. Patients in later stages of syphilis may present with nonspecific oral erosions or split, fissured papules of the oral commissures, which might be confused with cheilitis. Any concern for syphilis should prompt serologic testing rapid plasma reagin (RPR). Syphilis is treated with penicillin; the duration depends on the stage. The presence of oral lesions does not change the management strategy.

Autoimmune Disease/Hypersensitivity

Autoimmune diseases and hypersensitivity include many of the dangerous, oral diagnoses that should not be missed, such as pemphigus vulgaris, Stevens-Johnson syndrome (SJS), Crohn disease, and leukemia.

Hypersensitivity reactions range from erythema multiforme to SJS/toxic epidural necrolysis (TEN). They can be induced by HSV and other infections or medications. Mucosal involvement is seen in all patients with SJS/TEN and erythema multiforme major and signifies more severe disease. Oral manifestations include erythema and edema of the lips along with painful intraoral bullae. The bullae rupture, leaving desquamated oral mucosa underneath that appears as an erosion. The diagnosis is based on the clinical findings. Treatment is primarily supportive and often requires admission to a burn unit. Corticosteroid use is controversial, with more evidence supporting the use of intravenous immunoglobulin (IVIG).[7,8]

Three diseases that are often confused are bullous pemphigoid, cicatricial pemphigoid, and pemphigus vulgaris. All three can have manifestations in the oral cavity. Bullous pemphigoid is an autoimmune blistering condition that primarily affects the skin but does have oral involvement in 30% to 50% of cases.[9] In contrast, cicatricial pemphigoid is primarily an oropharyngeal disease and rarely involves the skin. It is characterized by desquamative gingivitis and bullae. Significant ocular involvement may occur as well.[10] Diagnosis is confirmed by biopsy and serum testing for specific autoantibodies, which can be completed by oral surgery or dermatology. Pemphigus vulgaris is a more serious and potentially fatal condition. It typically presents with flaccid bullae that rupture easily, which means that the patient often presents with only erosions. The condition usually starts in the oropharynx and then spreads to involve the skin. Because the oral erosions are nonspecific in appearance, a high level of suspicion and urgent referral are mandatory to prevent the life-threatening complications seen with this disease. The mainstays of treatment of all of these bullous diseases are systemic steroids and immunomodulators such as methotrexate. Pemphigus vulgaris may require high-dose steroids or immune-modulating drugs, including IVIG.[11] These medications should be given in conjunction with consultation with a specialist.

Behçet disease is another autoimmune disease characterized by oral ulcers, genital ulcers, and uveitis. All three conditions may not be present in all patients. Oral lesions appear similar to aphthous ulcers but are more extensive and often multiple. Genital lesions occur in 75% of cases.[12] Treatment includes oral colchicine, topical anesthetics, and topical and/or systemic corticosteroids and should be given in conjunction with referral to rheumatology or dermatology.[13]

Aphthous ulcers (also known as canker sores) are among the most common oral lesions. They are painful, shallow, round ulcers with a grayish base. Unlike herpes labialis, they occur on nonkeratinized mucosa. They are neither infectious nor contagious. The cause is not well understood, but may be related to alterations in local cell-mediated immunity. Predisposing factors include stress, hormonal factors, infections, food hypersensitivity, immunocompromise, family history, and exposure to sodium lauryl sulfate (a common ingredient in toothpaste). The differential diagnosis includes many vitamin deficiencies, which may cause a similar picture. Aphthous ulcers are common in patients with inflammatory bowel disease.

Aphthous ulcers are categorized as minor, major, and herpetiform. Minor ulcers are the most common. They are smaller than 5 mm and heal within 10 to 14 days without scarring. Major ulcers are larger than 5 mm, can last for 6 weeks, and often scar. Herpetiform ulcers are characterized by multiple small clusters of pinpoint lesions lasting 7 to 10 days. Despite the name herpetiform, they are not caused by HSV.

The diagnosis is based on the clinical presentation; if there is any concern for malignancy, biopsy should be done. Treatment varies based on the category. Minor and herpetiform ulcers require only symptomatic treatment (magic mouthwash and oral pain medication). Major ulcers require at the least a topical steroid or amlexanox. Systemic steroids or immune-modulating drugs may be indicated and should be administered in consultation with dentistry/oral medicine or a rheumatologist.[14]

Many other systemic diseases can have nonspecific oral lesions as a predominant component. In addition to those discussed earlier, leukemia, systemic lupus erythematosus (SLE), Crohn disease, and ulcerative colitis all may present with oral lesions before the development of other symptoms. The presence of any oral lesion without a clear cause mandates referral to an oral surgeon or oral medicine specialist for diagnosis.

Malignancy

Oral cancer kills 1 American every hour. Of the 36,000 patients who will be diagnosed with oral cancer this year, almost half will be dead in 5 years.[15] This poor prognosis does not result from the inherent lethality of the disease; most oral cancer is curable if it is found while it is small enough to be resected with clean margins. However, many cases are discovered because of their metastases (often to lymph nodes in the neck) instead of their primary location. Screening for cancer is not a routine part of the job of emergency physicians. However, the reality is that emergency physicians may be the only health care providers who look in patients' mouths, particularly the patients who are most at risk: those who heavily abuse tobacco and alcohol. When performing an oral examination in response to a patient's specific complaint, there is an obligation to inform the patient about any lesion that raises concern and to document the finding.

Almost all oral cancers are squamous cell carcinomas. Most of them are caused by concurrent tobacco and alcohol use. Heavy smokers and drinkers have a 35-fold increased risk of developing oral cancer.[16] Diagnosing oral cancer based on the appearance of a lesion is difficult because there is no pathognomonic form. A lesions that is exophytic or ulcerated can also be a papule, plaque, or erosion. Cancerous lesions can be painful, but most are painless (and therefore unnoticed by the patient). Any persistent lesion is cancer until proved otherwise by biopsy. Any patient with a lesion that cannot be diagnosed definitively by its clinical appearance must be referred to a specialist for work-up.

Benign Conditions

Tori can occur on either the mandible or the maxilla and do not indicate a pathologic condition; they are a bony growth that is a variant of normal anatomy. However, when patients discover them, they might come to the ED because they are concerned about having a tumor. Tori are present at birth. In the mandible, they are almost always bilateral, and they generally appear on the midline of the palate on the maxilla. They are not painful. As variants of normal anatomy, they do not require intervention.

Mucoceles are soft, translucent or blue, fluid-filled papules or nodules. They are mucus extravasation cysts, typically caused by (minor) trauma to small salivary ducts. No specific treatment is warranted. Ranulas are large mucoceles on the floor of the mouth. They most commonly arise from the sublingual gland but can also come from the submandibular gland. Surgery may be required to correct them. Incision and drainage or aspiration are ineffective, because the cyst will recur unless it is marsupialized.[17]

A fibroma is a smooth, mucosa-colored, exophytic mass. It is caused by reactive connective tissue hyperplasia induced by a chronic irritant (such as a broken tooth or oral piercing). In rare cases, they undergo malignant transformation, so excisional biopsy is usually recommended.

A lipoma is a benign tumor composed of adipose tissue. It is soft, mobile, and painless. For lipomas that occur anywhere else, treatment is not necessary unless they are painful or interfere with mastication. If they are large or continue to grow, biopsy may be considered to rule out malignancy.

Neurofibromas are benign nerve sheath tumors. They are often linked with genetic disease, such as neurofibromatosis or multiple endocrine neoplasia, type 2B. They can occur anywhere in the body, including the oral cavity. Resection is generally not indicated unless they are painful or interfere with mastication.

WHITE OR YELLOW LESIONS

Many white or yellow lesions have clear infectious or benign neoplastic causes, whereas the cause of others is idiopathic.

Infectious causes are primarily viral or fungal pathogens. Koplik spots are pathognomonic lesions for measles. They are rarely seen because of widespread vaccination. They appear as small, white lesions on the buccal mucosa near the Stensen duct. They should be associated with the other symptoms of measles. Treatment is supportive, and patients should be isolated as soon as the disease is suspected.

Oral hairy leukoplakia is caused by the Epstein-Barr virus (EBV) and is seen almost exclusively in patients with HIV. It appears as white plaque, often with filamentous projections. It occurs primarily on the tongue but may also be seen on the buccal mucosa. It is not painful and cannot be scraped off. Treatment is not necessary unless it is causing symptoms or is of cosmetic concern to the patient. The most effective treatment is to improve the immune system with highly active antiretroviral therapy, but specific treatment such as systemic antivirals (acyclovir, valacyclovir, or famciclovir) or local treatment (podophyllin, retinoic acid, or cryotherapy) can be used as well.[18]

Oral candidiasis is a fungal infection. It appears as thick, white deposits on nonkeratinized mucosa. It can be scraped off, often leaving an inflamed/bleeding base. It is generally painful and irritating to the patient. Topical therapy is usually effective, although relapses are common in immunocompromised patients. Options include nystatin suspension, nystatin troches, or clotrimazole troches for 7 to 14 days.[19] Nystatin suspension is cheapest, but clotrimazole troches are best tolerated.[20] Systemic fluconazole should be given to patients with recurrent moderate infection. Esophageal candidiasis does not respond to topical therapy alone.

Leukoplakia presents as white patches or plaques of the oral mucosa that cannot be scraped off. This appearance is caused by hyperplasia of the squamous epithelium. The cause may be repetitive mechanical trauma caused by oral piercings, a broken tooth, or an orthodontic appliance. This repetitive trauma can cause hyperplasia of the tissue surrounding the offending object. However, leukoplakia can also be precancerous, particularly lesions that have an erythematous component. Many of these lesions are associated with human papillomavirus (HPV),[21] so appropriate referral for biopsy is warranted.

Lichen planus typically appears as lacelike white patches on the buccal mucosa, but it can also present as erosions on the gingival margin or on the tongue. Lesions are generally painful. The cause is not clear; it can be a chronic disease by itself or associated with drug abuse, hepatitis C, or autoimmune conditions such as SLE. Patients with lichen planus are at increased risk for oral cancer. Treatment in the ED is based on symptoms (pain control), but follow-up for biopsy is imperative.

Fordyce spots are benign neoplasms of sebaceous glands. They are white to yellow discrete papules, 1 to 2 mm in diameter. They usually occur on the vermillion/buccal mucosal border. No treatment is necessary, although they can be removed with laser treatment if they are of cosmetic concern.

BROWN OR BLACK LESIONS

Malignant melanoma may present in the oral cavity. Its appearance is similar to melanoma anywhere else on the body. It is difficult to distinguish melanoma from the other benign brown and black lesions described later. In most cases, diagnosis depends on biopsy. Treatment is surgical and similar to that of melanoma at other body locations. However, the prognosis is often worsened by a delay in diagnosis.

Melanosis is a benign condition, similar to freckles. It is common in dark-skinned individuals. It can generally be distinguished from melanoma by the diffuse pattern of small pigmented areas, as opposed to the (generally) single, large lesion of melanoma.

Oral melanotic macules are also benign lesions. They may be more darkly pigmented than the other lesions discussed in this article. Oral melanotic macules are often found on the lips or the oral mucosa and are typically symmetric with sharp borders. They present in adulthood. They frequently require biopsy to distinguish between this condition and malignancy.[22,23]

Amalgam tattoos are blue-black macules seen in the oral mucosa adjacent to an amalgam dental filling. They occur during the process of restoring the tooth, when a small fragment of the amalgam is embedded in the soft tissue. Their appearance is similar to that of oral melanomas, so if there is any doubt to the diagnosis, biopsy is recommended.

LESIONS OF THE TONGUE

Some oral lesions affect only the tongue. Among these are black hairy tongue and geographic tongue.

Black hairy tongue is a benign condition characterized by elongated discolored (usually brown to black) filiform papillae on the dorsal surface of the tongue. This condition is not painful. It often causes bad breath. It is not related to hairy leukoplakia and is typically not infectious, although it may be superimposed on candidal infection. It can be associated with antibiotic use. In most patients, it is caused by poor oral hygiene. Treatment is to improve oral hygiene, paying special attention to brushing the tongue.

Geographic tongue is also aptly known as benign migratory glossitis. It presents as erythematous patches on the dorsal tongue with circumferential white polycyclic borders. The tongue lesions can change location, pattern, and size within minutes. Geographic tongue is usually asymptomatic but may cause burning and discomfort. Its cause is unknown, and the condition tends to be recurrent. It often is triggered by specific foods or substances. There is no specific treatment other than patient reassurance.

CHEILITIS

Cheilitis involves the lips. Angular chelitis is characterized by erythema and scaling of the lips. As the name suggests, it is usually located at the corners of the mouth. It is caused by retinoids, environmental exposure, allergies, vitamin deficiencies, and lip licking. In most cases, it is an entirely benign condition, treated by avoidance of the irritant and use of moisturizing lip balm. If vitamin deficiency is suspected, consider further work-up. Secondary infection, both bacterial and fungal, occurs rarely and should be treated when present.

In contrast, actinic cheilitis is not benign and can occur anywhere along the lips at the vermillion border. It appears as a scaly, whitish discoloration, sometimes surrounded by erythematous ulceration. It is usually related to sun exposure and/or tobacco use and is a precursor to invasive squamous cell carcinoma. Referral for excisional biopsy is mandatory.

SUMMARY

Oral lesions can be challenging to diagnose in the ED. A wide spectrum of pathologic conditions can present in the mouth, ranging from local and benign to systemic and deadly. The job of the emergency physician is to recognize the few diseases that require immediate intervention and to ensure appropriate follow-up for the rest. Recognition of lesions can be aided by the use of a color-scheme classification. For many patients in the United States, the ED may be their only point of contact with the health care system. Recognition of potential oral malignancy (and other dangerous conditions) followed by appropriate referral can be lifesaving.

REFERENCES

1. Negrin RS, Bedard JF, Toljanic JA. Oral toxicity associated with chemotherapy. UpToDate; 2011. Accessed January 10, 2012.
2. Goldstein BG, Goldstein AO. Oral lesions. Available at: www.uptodate.com. Accessed February 21, 2012.
3. Gilbert SC. Management and prevention of recurrent herpes labialis in immunocompetent patients. Herpes 2007;14:56–61.
4. Rooney JF, Straus SE, Mannix ML, et al. Oral acyclovir to suppress frequently recurrent herpes labialis. A double-blind, placebo-controlled trial. Ann Intern Med 1993;118:268–72.

5. Baker D, Eisen D. Valacyclovir for prevention of recurrent herpes labialis: 2 double-blind, placebo-controlled studies. Cutis 2003;71:239–42.

6. Nichols CM, Flaitz CM, Hicks MJ. Treating Kaposi's lesions in the HIV-infected patient. J Am Dent Assoc 1993;124:78–84.

7. Schneck J, Fagot JP, Sekula P, et al. Effects of treatments on the mortality of Stevens-Johnson syndrome and toxic epidermal necrolysis: a retrospective study on patients included in the prospective EuroSCAR Study. J Am Acad Dermatol 2008;58:33–40.

8. French LE, Trent JT, Kerdel FA. Use of intravenous immunoglobulin in toxic epidermal necrolysis and Stevens-Johnson syndrome: our current understanding. Int Immunopharmacol 2006;6:543–9.

9. Greenberg MS, Ship JA, Glick M, editors. Burket's oral medicine. 11th edition. Hamilton (Ontario): BC Decker; 2008.

10. Ahmed AR, Kurgis BS, Rogers RS. Cicatricial pemphigoid. J Am Acad Dermatol 1991;24:987–1001.

11. Zeina B, Sakka N, Mansoor S. Pemphigus vulgaris. Updated: July 28, 2011. Available at: http://emedicine.medscape.com/article/1064187-overview. Accessed February 21, 2012.

12. O'Duffy JD. Behcet's syndrome. In: Schumacher HR, editor. Primer on the rheumatic diseases. 10th edition. Atlanta (GA): Arthritis Foundation; 1993. p. 307–8.

13. Sakane T, Takeno M, Suzuki N, et al. Behçet's disease. N Engl J Med 1999;341: 1284–91.

14. Altenburg A, Abdel-Naser MB, Seeber H, et al. Practical aspects of management of recurrent aphthous stomatitis. J Eur Acad Dermatol Venereol 2007;21:1019–26.

15. American Cancer Society. Cancer facts & figures 2009. Atlanta (GA): American Cancer Society; 2009.

16. Blot WJ, McLaughlin JK, Winn DM, et al. Smoking and drinking in relation to oral and pharyngeal cancer. Cancer Res 1988;48:3282–7.

17. Isaacson GC. Congenital anomalies of the jaw, mouth, oral cavity, and pharynx. Available at: www.uptodate.com. Accessed January 10, 2012.

18. Kozyreva O. Hairy leukoplakia. Updated December 2, 2009. Available at: http://emedicine.medscape.com/article/279269-overview. Accessed December 14, 2011.

19. Patton LL, Bonito AJ, Shugars DA. A systematic review of the effectiveness of antifungal drugs for the prevention and treatment of oropharyngeal candidiasis in HIV-positive patients. Oral Surg Oral Med Oral Pathol Oral Radiol Endod 2001;92:170–9.

20. Klotz SA. Oropharyngeal candidiasis: a new treatment option. Clin Infect Dis 2006;42:1187–8.

21. Cianfriglia F, Di Gregorio DA, Cianfriglia C, et al. Incidence of human papillomavirus infection in oral leukoplakia. Indications for a viral aetiology. J Exp Clin Cancer Res 2006;25:21–8.

22. Eisen D, Voorhees JJ. Oral melanoma and other pigmented lesions of the oral cavity. J Am Acad Dermatol 1991;24:527–37.

23. Kaugars GE, Heise AP, Riley WT, et al. Oral melanotic macules. A review of 353 cases. Oral Surg Oral Med Oral Pathol 1993;76:59–61.

Dental and Related Infections

Alan Hodgdon, MD, MBA

KEYWORDS

- Intraoral infection • Periapical abscess • Periodontal abscess
- Necrotizing ulcerative gingivitis (NUG) • Ludwig's angina • Facial cellulitis

KEY POINTS

- Emergency physicians should be comfortable treating most dental and related infections.
- Failing to refer patients for routine dental care after noting poor oral hygiene and dental caries is a common pitfall. Tooth loss is often preventable when follow-up dental care is made available and used. In addition, recent studies have linked dental health to overall long-term health status.
- Another pitfall is failing to drain an abscess cavity, when one is noted, in favor of antibiotic therapy.
- The potential critical nature of a deep space infection of the face or neck should be recognized, such as Ludwig's angina or facial cellulitis.
- Adequate analgesia should be provided for intraoral procedures, such as incision and drainage. This analgesia can be provided via supraperiosteal injection by the individual tooth or inferior alveolar nerve block for the lower teeth, with a long-acting anesthetic such as bupivacaine.

INTRODUCTION

Pain in the jaw and other facial structures is a common presenting complaint in most emergency departments. It is the job of the emergency physician to determine which of these complaints demands immediate therapy and which can be ameliorated until a dentist or oral-maxillofacial surgeon (OMFS) is available. Most dental-related problems can be treated with simple therapies and are within the realm of well-trained emergency physicians. Some of the more important dental-related problems are related to infections originating in the tooth that then spread to adjacent tissues, including gingiva, surrounding soft tissues of the face and neck, or to the alveolar bone of the jaw.[1]

As with all good medicine, a thorough medical history and review of systems should be obtained before oral examination begins, providing the airway does not require intervention. Although emergency clinicians are concerned with acute disease, many chronic diseases, from clotting disorders to cancers, can manifest with oral

Department of Emergency Medicine, University of Pittsburgh School of Medicine, 230 McKee Place, Suite 500, Pittsburgh, PA 15213, USA
E-mail address: hodgdona@upmc.edu

Emerg Med Clin N Am 31 (2013) 465–480
http://dx.doi.org/10.1016/j.emc.2013.01.007
0733-8627/13/$ – see front matter Published by Elsevier Inc.

emed.theclinics.com

disorders and these should not be ignored. A basic review of the patient's medical history can reveal information important in weighing risk/benefit in the use of medications and treatment options. For example, a history of splenectomy, neutropenia, sepsis, regurgitant heart valve, recent dental work, mandible fracture, and other medical history are important details that potentially influence not only the examination but the treatment options. For example, the risk of serious bacterial infection must be weighed against the risk of anaphylaxis and other side effects when antibiotics are prescribed for oral infections. Because manipulation of the oral cavity often causes transient bacteremia, those patients who should have prophylaxis with antibiotics should be identified before doing invasive procedures of the mouth. A good history helps identify these individuals.

This article presents a brief overview of infections associated with the oral cavity and supporting structures, beginning with the most common and superficial. Understanding and dealing with these in day-to-day practice makes it easier to diagnose and treat sicker patients whose disorders are related to, but not confined within, the oral cavity.

TOOTH ANATOMY

To understand how an apical abscess develops and how other common tooth disorders cause pain, it is important to briefly review some points about tooth anatomy. The enamel is the hard outer surface of the tooth. Intact enamel is white and shiny. Although this appearance can be dulled by plaque and tooth staining, it can usually be ascertained whether the enamel is intact by looking closely at the surface of the tooth. Besides plaque disguising the enamel of the tooth, long-term plaque supports the growth of organisms that destroy enamel, and this is the underlying disorder of dental caries, so significant plaque warrants referral for routine care.

Under the enamel lies the dentin. It is off-yellow in color, and sensate. If the dentin is exposed, it becomes inflamed and painful. In addition, unprotected dentin is sensitive to infection because it is composed of porous microtubules that connect directly to the pulp cavity. In the pulp cavity lie the nerve and blood supplies of the tooth and so the dentin is an important structure. When it is exposed by either caries or trauma, it should be covered. This reduces pain and lessens the chance for infection to track along the microtubules to the dental pulp. It also lessens the chances of pulp necrosis.

Although there is a specific tooth numbering system, the more practical method is just to name the tooth involved, keeping in mind the general dental formula. The dental formula states that the mouth can be divided into 4 quadrants, each having the following teeth from the midline: central incisor, lateral incisor, canine, 2 premolars, and 3 molars (the last or third molar is the wisdom tooth). Using this simple formula, all teeth can be properly identified when documenting disorders and discussing them with specialists.

ORAL EXAMINATION

Emergency department management is based on a thorough history and a meticulous physical examination of the face, mouth, and neck. If the patient appears acutely ill, airway assessment should take precedence. There are several algorithms regarding potentially difficult airways, but, even without touching the patient, an evaluation of the size and mobility of the neck, the interincisor distance, and the appearance of the submental area can be done to see if this is likely to be a difficult intubation.[2]

If the airway is not in any danger of occluding, proceed to the patient's general appearance, concentrating on facial symmetry. Evaluate for facial edema, localized external areas of tenderness, erythema, and obvious lesions. The lymph nodes in the neck, including those in the submandibular and preauricular regions are palpated. Then proceed to examine the mouth.

It is best to evaluate the mouth with a tongue blade in each hand, with good lighting from either a headlamp or a good overhead light. Both hands should be free to feel in the mouth and hold the tongue blades. After you have gloved and are holding a tongue blade in each hand, ask the patient to open his or her mouth. Evaluate first for trismus, which is noted almost immediately by the inability to fully open the mouth. The inter-incisor distance can be objectively measured by the distance between the maxillary and mandibular central incisors. A normal measurement is anything greater than 35 mm (approximately the width of 2 adult fingers). Measurements less than 30 mm (trismus) make intraoral examination more difficult and ultimate airway management more problematic. This distance can usually be estimated by the ability of the patient to open the mouth, but, if this looks difficult or impaired in any way, measure this distance. When mouth opening is limited by pain not associated with temporomandib-ular joint disorder, it usually indicates infection in the muscles of mastication, and is an indication for a more in-depth examination.[3–5] According to Christian,[6] writing about oromaxillofacial infections, "The hallmark of infection in any or all of the secondary spaces of the mandible (the masticator space) and by extension, the deep neck spaces, is trismus."

Proceeding from the outside in (labial mucosa), and from the anterior of the mouth posteriorly, evaluate the soft tissue structures for abnormality. Do this first before examining the teeth, because most tooth disorders cause problems with the surrounding gingiva. Begin at the inferior lip, looking for erosions, state of dentition, erythema, abscess, and for areas of inflammation. Proceeding to the posterior mucosa, evaluate the posterior oropharynx, then the tongue. Palpate along the base of the vestibule looking for signs of swelling, tenderness, or purulence. After eval-uating these supporting structures, evaluate the teeth, focusing on areas noted in the initial visual inspection or by evaluating areas of pain as described by the patient. There are ways to use heat or cold to stress the nerves of the teeth, but the percussion test works best, is simple, and is sensitive.[7] Percussing the occlusal surface of a tooth that has an inflamed nerve usually elicits pain. When tenderness is elicited on exam-ination in an area, be specific (ie, try to determine which tooth the disorder is coming from, rather than just a region). This method helps in determining whether the tooth disorder is old or new and helps guide therapy. In most cases, old dead teeth are usually not markedly tender, because the root of the tooth is already necrotic. It is acutely infected and inflamed teeth that tend to be painful.

After the gingiva and tooth structures are evaluated with the tongue blades, repeat the examination with a focus on the area of complaint, carefully identifying the disorder found. This repeat percussion and examination helps localize the disorder. Look closely at the involved tooth surfaces, the gingiva associated with the suspect tooth, and attempt to move the tooth. Loose teeth and recession of the gingival structures indicate advanced periodontal disease. Palpate the tongue and floor of the mouth and examine the mucosa for lesions.

The patient should have a reproducible examination, and not simply complain of generalized areas of pain. Although it is helpful to know that old areas of decay are not sensitive to percussion or palpation, caution is needed. An old area of decay is subjective and some necrotic-appearing areas can be painful. The reason for this is that the pulp in multirooted teeth does not die at an even rate. It is possible to have a dead root in a multirooted tooth like a molar, but to have 2 or more roots that are still viable and painful. This principle is important because of the issue of narcotic overuse and abuse, which has increased in recent years, and toothache is a common presentation of this problem. Although there is no doubt that oxycodone and hydrocodone are effective pain medications, nonsteroidal antiinflammatory drugs (NSAIDs) are more effective in general for pain in the oral cavity than in most other body locations, and are the drugs of choice for pain in this region. This effectiveness has been shown repeatedly, not only with the older medications such as aspirin and ibuprofen but with newer NSAIDs such as celecoxib, etoricoxib, and rofecoxib, with or without adjunctive medications such as acetaminophen.[8–19] NSAIDs may not only work better with respect to lowering pain scores, they may do this for a longer period than even a significant dose of acetaminophen with codeine (600/60 mg). In a study by Malmstrom and colleagues,[20] the duration of analgesic effect, defined as median time to rescue medication use, was greater than 24 hours for etoricoxib, 20.8 hours for naproxen sodium, 3.6 hours for acetaminophen/codeine, and 1.6 hours for placebo.

In the book *Pain Management: Part 1: Managing Acute and Postoperative Dental Pain*, Becker[21] concludes a discussion about NSAID use: "The nonopioid analgesics include acetaminophen (APAP) and the nonsteroidal anti-inflammatory drugs (NSAIDs). The analgesic efficacy of these agents is typically underestimated. This is unfortunate because they generally are equivalent or superior to opioids for managing musculoskeletal pain, and they produce a lower incidence of side effects, including the potential for abuse."

In addition to better and more prolonged pain control with NSAIDS, a reduction in narcotic use can be seen when NSAIDS are prescribed instead of narcotics as part of odontalgia guidelines. In a study by Ma and colleagues,[22] guidelines for both patients and providers in the community were instituted. For providers, there were prescribing guidelines and for patients, there were guidelines about appropriate visits and other community resources for dental problems. About 6000 visits for odontalgia were studied before and after the institution of the program. The proportion of visits for odontalgia decreased after guideline implementation from 4.3% to 3.1%. The proportion of patients with return visits decreased from 19.8% to 9.2% and the proportion of patients filling narcotic prescriptions for odontalgia decreased from 29.6% to 9.5%. The implementation of guidelines is a reasonable way to conserve emergency resources for those complaints more emergent in nature, and to reduce inappropriate narcotic use as well. When narcotics are prescribed for oral pain, a limited supply is appropriate. In addition, most patients who need a narcotic do well with an NSAID for day use and a narcotic at night.

The use of long-acting anesthetics such as bupivacaine has also been shown to be beneficial in controlling odontalgic pain, especially when combined with the use of an NSAID. A supraperiosteal injection placed in the region of the affected tooth provides long-term pain control and decreases the need for narcotic analgesia, even after the anesthetic affect has abated. Injectable anesthetics should be considered in any patient with odontogenic pain.

With the history and physical examination conducted in an organized manner, the diseases described later can be diagnosed and appropriate treatment begun. Disorders are divided into those of the teeth versus those of the supporting structures of the teeth.

DISEASES OF THE TEETH
Dental Caries

Dental caries, or tooth decay, is the oldest and most common cause of toothache seen in the emergency department and the most common cause of tooth loss worldwide.[23]

This is not an acute process, but eventually the pain increases until often the patient cannot take it any longer. Pain is associated with exposure of the dentin and, in advanced cases, with irritation of the pulp called pulpitis. Associated periodontal disease, if severe, may contribute to the pain. The process consists of a complex interaction of at-risk teeth, bacteria (mostly *Streptococcus mutans*), and the proper acidic environment. As such, caries of the teeth, as well as periodontal diseases in general, are bacterial in nature. Plaque is associated with this process, and its buildup and lack of proper dental care are largely responsible for this preventable disease.

The patient with deep caries usually complains of dull pain, often exacerbated by hot or cold foods. Percussion of the involved tooth and evaluation of the associated mucosa helps determine appropriate pain medication before referral. Unless pulpitis or other disorders are evident on examination, antibiotics are not indicated.[24] Definitive therapy involves excavation and filling of the decayed areas by a general dentist.

Pulpitis

Pulpitis is inflammation of the confined structures of the pulp cavity, usually caused by associated infection. The most common symptom is pain, because the vascular and nerve bundle are in the pulp cavity. The patient complains of severe pain, often throbbing and shooting in character. The pain is exacerbated by thermal changes. The most common cause of these infections is extension of infection from dental caries, but pulpitis can occur from trauma or chemical irritation as well. Pulpitis can be acute and reversible, but chronic, irreversible pulpitis can also occur. In chronic pulpitis, pain is less intense and less temperature sensitive. Definitive treatment of irreversible pulpitis involves excavation and filling of the underlying dental caries, and usually a root canal. Root canal therapy removes the structures of the root, specifically the nerve and vascular bundle, and thereby helps solve several serious tooth disorders without the need for tooth extraction.

Periapical Abscess

When dental caries are left unchecked for prolonged periods the infection tracks to the pulp cavity, causing pulpitis. Over time, this is followed by extension of the infection to the cancellous bone of the dentoalveolar ridge. Here the infection usually tracks toward the surface of the bone and can be both seen and palpated (**Fig. 1**). The clinician must look for this disorder, because it is readily treatable with incision and drainage (I & D) by experienced emergency clinicians or by a dental consultant. Anesthesia via supraperiosteal injection is performed by injecting a small volume of anesthetic in the soft mucobuccal fold near the root of the tooth, and I & D can be performed easily under this simple local anesthesia. For further details of intraoral drainage procedures, the reader

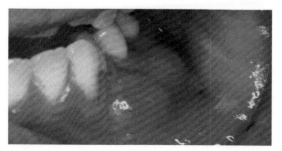

Fig. 1. Periapical abscess.

is referred to common emergency procedures texts.[25] Drainage of this infection can prevent the further tracking of the infection to other areas of the face and neck. I & D is the treatment of choice until definitive treatment can be completed, because antibiotics do not penetrate well into the area of abscess.

After I & D, and after any oral procedure performed, the patient should swish and spit with warm salt solution until the spit is clear and a quick reexamination of the mouth can be performed. An antibiotic should be prescribed to decrease the ongoing infection in the pulp, making definitive care more manageable by the dental consultant. The antibiotic of choice is penicillin (Penn VK 500 mg 4 times a day), or clindamycin 300 mg 4 times a day. Erythromycin or another macrolide is also an acceptable choice. The patient should be given instructions for a follow-up visit with a dental consultant within 2 to 3 days.

A few comments should be made here about the use of antibiotics in intraoral infections. Although general antibiotic resistance has been increasing and some OMFSs recommend amoxicillin/clavulanate instead of either penicillin VK or simple amoxicillin, data support the general principle of first-line therapy with simple, inexpensive antibiotics when possible.[26] The rationale for expanded coverage is that approximately 34% of *Prevotella* strains are β-lactamase producing, possibly leading to treatment failures, which is worrisome in cases of deeper space infections or infections at high risk, such as facial cellulitis or Ludwig's angina, for which amoxicillin/clavulanate, clindamycin, and metronidazole are better choices.[27]

Definitive treatment of periapical abscess involves either extraction of the tooth or excavation and filling of the underlying denal caries followed by a root canal. The choice of definitive procedure depends on the health of the involved teeth and supporting structures, anticipated compliance of the patient, and the resources available. Root canal therapy requires a patient who can comply with more than 1 office visit and follow instructions. In austere environments (ie, third world locations) or with noncompliant patients, tooth extraction is the most expeditious and probably the best method to definitively deal with this disorder.

A common pitfall of periapical abscess is to try to avoid I & D of the abscess by simply treating the patient with antibiotics. This error is often related to the experience or knowledge of the emergency physician, and puts the patient at risk for extension of the infection and delayed pain relief.

PERIODONTAL DISEASES

Periodontal disease is often thought of as gum disease. The periodontium consists of the supporting structures of the gingiva, periodontal ligament, and alveolar bone and is a group of diseases. The 2 most important in terms of numbers are gingivitis and periodontitis, both of which are discussed later.

The most common cause of periodontal disease is poor dental hygiene, with the subsequent buildup of plaque, resulting in both dental caries and potentially periodontal disease. As with dental caries, bacterial interplay with susceptible structures precipitates the inflammation and degeneration of the structures affected. Many systemic diseases are also associated with periodontal diseases, the most common being poorly controlled insulin or non–insulin dependent diabetes, human immunodeficiency virus infection, and cardiovascular diseases. In addition, hormonal factors and drug reactions can also cause specific types of periodontal diseases. Neither gingivitis nor periodontitis is by itself an emergency, but the complications of these diseases result in many emergency department visits each year, so a basic understanding of these processes is important.

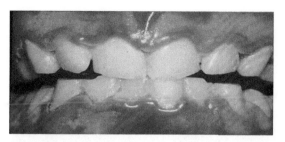

Fig. 2. Gingivitis.

Gingivitis

Gingivitis is a reversible inflammatory process of the gingiva, characterized by a change in the normal contour of the gingiva, with erythema, edema, and often discharge. Despite changes in the gingiva, the junctional epithelium that covers the inferior portion of the tooth is maintained intact and the tooth is not loosened. Treatment of gingivitis is local debridement to remove plaque, the causative factor. The underlying systemic disease should also be addressed when it is a contributing factor (**Fig. 2**).

Periodontitis

Periodontitis is an inflammatory condition that is no longer isolated to the gingiva and is not reversible. It is characterized by loss of attachment of the periodontal ligament and the bony support of the tooth. It is thought to represent an extension of gingivitis, although most areas of gingivitis do not transition to periodontitis. The destruction of these supporting structures of the tooth does not proceed in a steady manner, but seems to progress in bursts related to the interplay of several factors. In the elderly, periodontitis is still a significant cause of tooth loss. Evidence of periodontitis should be noted on examination and referred to a dentist for evaluation and treatment.

Periodontal Abscess

When periodontitis is advanced, the associated bone loss can result in localized pockets forming around the tooth. These pockets can become infected, resulting in pain, erythema, and frank abscess. This type of abscess differs from the periapical abscess because the tooth may still be healthy and no caries need be present (**Fig. 3**).

Initial treatment consists of local anesthesia, usually a supraperiosteal injection, followed by I & D by either the emergency physician or dental consultant. Antibiotics are usually not indicated because the underlying tooth is not affected, unless the area of abscess is extensive. The patient should be referred to a dentist for further management, which usually involves physical removal of all calculus buildup and curettage of the periodontal pocket.

Empiric use of amoxicillin or cephalexin after surgical treatment in deeper dentoalveolar abscess treatment has been shown to significantly reduce the duration of clinical symptoms in a study of acute odontogenic infections in comparison with surgical treatment alone.[28] Bacterial strains isolated in early stages of dentoalveolar abscess showed high sensitivity to amoxicillin and cephalexin. Duration of treatment can be limited. In a study of 188 patients with dentoalveolar abscess, a standard 3-day regimen of antibiotics was as effective as longer regimens, when associated with appropriate drainage.[29]

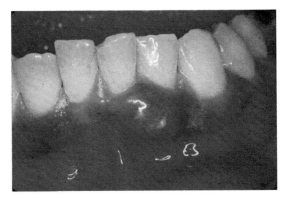

Fig. 3. Periodontal abscess.

Pericoronitis

Pericoronitis is inflammation, usually followed by infection, of the gingival tissue over-lying the crown of an impacted tooth. As the tooth attempts to erupt through this gingiva (operculum), the area becomes inflamed and secondarily infected. This process usually involves the wisdom teeth (third molars), and the severity can range from mild inflammation to a significant spreading facial infection. Often extraction of the maxillary third molar greatly improves the situation, because it is often the maxillary tooth that causes the trauma to the operculum covering the lower third molar, but the course of treatment can vary, therefore follow-up with dentists is required.

Emergency treatment is based on severity, but usually involves oral antibiotic administration of penicillin VK or clindamycin. Erythromycin or another macrolide is also an acceptable choice. Adequate pain medications should be given and urgent referral to an oral surgeon should be made. Definitive treatment usually involves extraction of the impacted tooth if the infection is severe.

Acute Herpetic Gingivostomatitis

This is an acute infection usually noted in early childhood. It represents the first infection with herpes and, as such, presents with a classic prodrome of illness, followed by lymphadenopathy and fever. The oral lesions are usually multiple, shallow, round, and discrete ulcers with a red halo of inflammation. The gingiva is usually inflamed and painful (**Figs. 4** and **5**).

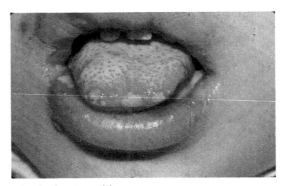

Fig. 4. Acute herpetic gingivostomatitis.

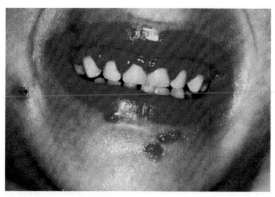

Fig. 5. Acute herpetic gingivostomatitis.

Acute treatment is symptomatic, ensuring control of fever and adequate hydration. A swizzle of equal parts viscous lidocaine, magnesium hydroxide and aluminum hydroxide, and diphenhydramine can be given for symptomatic relief of oral pain. Debacterol has been shown to speed healing and reduce pain of oral ulcers in diseases such as aphthous ulcers, and is fast replacing swizzle in most oral ulcer treatment.[30]

Necrotizing Ulcerative Gingivitis

Necrotizing ulcerative gingivitis (NUG), also called trench mouth or Vincent infection, is an intraoral infection characterized by erythema and hyperemia of the gingiva, fetid breath, bleeding gums, and friability of the mucosa. White plaques and areas of ulceration are usually evident and a pseudomembrane may be present, which bleeds with manipulation (**Figs. 6** and **7**).

Three specific clinical characteristics must be present to diagnose NUG: pain, interdental necrosis, and bleeding.[31] The pain is usually of rapid onset, which helps to distinguish this disorder from an autoimmune chronic disorder with similar but less severe and chronic symptoms.[32] Systemic symptoms are often present, such as fever, malaise, or dehydration.

The disease occurs mostly in teenagers, and is associated with factors such as malnutrition, smoking, stress, or poor personal hygiene. Such factors favor the proliferation of fusiform and spirochete bacteria responsible for the infection.

NUG is primarily treated with local mouth care. Options include gentle debridement of lesions with a cotton-tipped swab soaked with hydrogen peroxide, rinse with equal parts hydrogen peroxide (3%) and warm water every 2 to 3 hours, or chlorhexidine oral rinse twice daily. Antiseptic mouthwash such as chlorhexidine 0.12% decreases

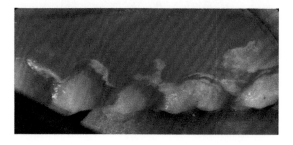

Fig. 6. NUG.

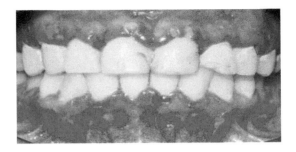

Fig. 7. NUG.

bacterial count and is effective when used in combination with good mouth care, rinses, brushing, and flossing.[33]

Antibiotics (metronidazole or penicillin) are indicated if systemic involvement is evident (ie, fever or lymphadenopathy) but the primary treatment is local mouth care. Pain medications should be prescribed so that proper mouth care can be done. Bony destruction can occur as a consequence of NUG, so follow-up needs to be arranged and compliance encouraged.[34]

Ludwig's Angina

There are many names for this serious deep tissue infection, but the most descriptive is submandibular cellulitis. This condition has been known for centuries and got its name from the hoarse voice, neck pain, and choking sensation it can cause.[35] Both its medical and surgical management can be complicated and it should be considered in any ill patient with ear, nose, and throat (ENT) or oromaxillofacial pain and swelling.[36] The diagnosis is not always obvious or clear-cut, partly because the anatomy in the region of the anterior neck is not well understood by most physicians and the edema and erythema that occur in this space can be diffuse and subtle. The key point to understand here is that the investing layer of the deep cervical fascia of the neck attaches to both the undersurface of the mandible and the hyoid bone. The lateral extension of this fascia forms the submandibular space, with the superior portion bounded by the floor of the mouth. As with all fascia, the nondistensible nature of this structure explains why swelling in this space is reflected by displacement of the floor of the mouth and elevation of the tongue, with little edema in the midline of the neck (**Figs. 8** and **9**).[37]

The most common cause of Ludwig's angina is dental infections, specifically involving the roots of the second and third mandibular molars, which are just superior

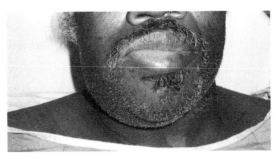

Fig. 8. Ludwig's angina.

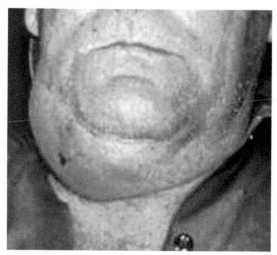

Fig. 9. Ludwig's angina.

to this submandibular space and contiguous with it. The next most common cause is extension from an upper airway infection, such as peritonsillar abscess.[38] There are other uncommon causes related to other ENT lesions and infections.[39]

Most significant infections in the mouth are polymicrobial and Ludwig's angina is no exception. Common organisms include a mixture of aerobic and anaerobic organisms such as streptococci, staphylococci, and *Fusobacterium*. As such, intravenous (IV) ampicillin or a β-lactam penicillin with metronidazole is recommended as empiric therapy, with clindamycin commonly used for patients who are allergic to penicillin.

Severe airway complication and resultant death are the main complications of this disease and can occur rapidly. Early recognition and expert management are therefore of utmost importance with careful attention to the precipitous nature of the airway if the disease worsens acutely. Other causes of death include mediastinitis and sepsis.[40]

Patients with Ludwig's angina can present from the early stages, at which there is just submandibular swelling and minimal erythema, to those whose airway is endangered from tongue elevation, facial swelling, severe trismus, and a tender swollen neck. Emergency physicians must be aware of the potential for bad outcomes along this spectrum and pursue a thorough examination and often computed tomography (CT) of the neck to evaluate the extent of the disease. If the airway appears to be tenuous, a multidisciplinary approach with anesthesia, OMFS, ENT, and critical care personnel is favored.[41,42]

In early cases in which the airway is not involved, close observation without acute airway intervention can be pursued, usually by admission to the OMFS or ENT service and monitoring in a critical care or step-down unit of the hospital. IV antibiotics are provided and often a tracheostomy tray is situated at the bedside. Frequent reexamination by specialists detects any worsening of the patient's airway and, if this occurs, the patient is taken to the operating room for definitive airway therapy. This therapy usually consists of either endoscopically assisted nasotracheal intubation or tracheostomy under local anesthesia. With this management scheme, most patients can be managed with either observation and IV antibiotics or intubation with antibiotics.

In a 9-year study of 29 cases of Ludwig's angina, 21 patients were treated with observation, 7 were intubated with fiberoptic assistance, and 1 required local tracheostomy. There were no deaths in this study, which compares favorably with prior studies in which the disease was either not diagnosed immediately or not managed by appropriate specialists, in which morbidity and mortality were higher.[43]

Most of the studies on this disease, such as the one discussed earlier, are from large teaching hospitals where many of these cases are managed. These tertiary hospitals have a multitude of resources immediately available, including specialists who have managed many of these cases. In smaller hospitals with fewer resources and doubt about safe management, surgical drainage may be a safer option for Ludwig's angina unless the extent of cellulitis is limited or the size of the abscess is small.

As suggested earlier, the diagnosis is not clear-cut in many patients because of anatomic considerations of the anterior neck. Sometimes an abscess can be missed because of induration and inflammation of the submandibular glands, which can be confusing. In these cases, CT of the neck can help to decide the extension of the infection, whether it is localized or a more generalized cellulitis, and guide therapy for both the specialist and the emergency physician. Anterior visceral space involvement and diabetes mellitus were the most important predictive factors in a recent diagnostic model, in which logistic regression analysis also confirmed bilateral submandibular swelling and other comorbidities as risk factors for the development of Ludwig's angina.[44] In a recent study, amoxicillin-clavulanate was the most active antibiotic against all species tested, followed by metronidazole in the case of anaerobes.[45]

Facial Cellulitis

Facial cellulitis must be treated more aggressively than cellulitis in other body areas because of the morbidity and mortality of complications, which include cavernous sinus thrombosis and possible extension of the cellulitis to the brain. Most patients with facial cellulitis are admitted for IV antibiotics, especially when there is significant facial involvement or systemic symptoms such as fever. Most facial cellulitis is caused by extension of infection from the oral cavity, whereas acute sinusitis accounts for most of the remainder of causes. Because each upper central incisor drains bilaterally, they are of more concern when they become infected, although the maxillary molars are the most common origin of facial cellulitis (**Figs. 10** and **11**).[46]

In children, it is important to distinguish facial cellulitis from buccal cellulitis, but the era of systemic buccal cellulitis in the United States is almost gone with the advent of *Haemophilus influenzae* type b vaccine. The organisms responsible for facial cellulitis in adults are usually mixed flora. In a recent study of cultures taken at surgical drainage, 19% of the samples contained only aerobic organisms, 36% only anaerobic organisms, and 45% contained mixed aerobic and anaerobic flora. *Streptococcus*

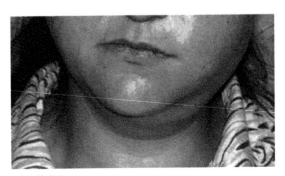

Fig. 10. Facial/buccal cellulitis.

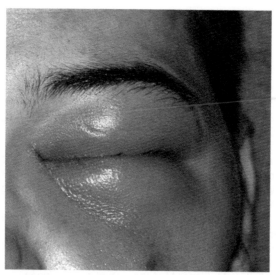

Fig. 11. Facial/buccal cellulitis.

was the most frequently isolated aerobic bacteria, noted in 65% of infections. Anaerobic bacteria accounted for 62% of isolates and the most frequently isolated were *Prevotella* spp, in 55% of cases.[47]

SUMMARY

Emergency physicians should be comfortable treating most dental and related infections. The most common pitfalls are:

1. Failing to refer patients for routine dental care after noting poor oral hygiene and dental caries. Tooth loss is often preventable when follow-up dental care is made available and used. In addition, recent studies have linked dental health to overall long-term health status.
2. Failing to drain an abscess cavity, when one is noted, in favor of antibiotic therapy.
3. Failing to recognize the potential critical nature of a deep infection of the face or neck, such as Ludwig's angina.
4. Failing to provide adequate analgesia via supraperiosteal injection with a long-acting anesthetic such as bupivacaine.

REFERENCES

1. Trivedy C, Kodate N, Ross A, et al. Attitudes and awareness of emergency department (ED) physicians towards the management of common dentofacial emergencies. Dent Traumatol 2012;28(2):121–6.
2. Vissers RJ, Gibbs MA. The high-risk airway. Emerg Med Clin North Am 2010; 28(1):203–17, ix–x.
3. Placko G, Bellot-Samson V, Brunet S, et al. Normal mouth opening in the adult French population. Rev Stomatol Chir Maxillofac 2005;106(5):267–71.
4. Reynolds SC, Chow AW. Severe soft tissue infections of the head and neck: a primer for critical care physicians. Lung 2009;187(5):271–9.
5. Sohail A, Amjad A. The range of inter-incisal opening among university students of Ajman, UAE. Pak Oral Dental J 2011;31(1):37.

6. Christian JM. Odontogenic infections. In: Flint PW, Haughey BH, editors. Cummings Otolaryngology-Head & Neck Surgery. 5th edition. Philadelphia: Mosby Elsevier; 2010. p. 185–6.

7. Chapter 6. In: Torabinejad M, Walton RE, editors. Endodontics: principles and practice. Philadelphia: Elsevier Health Sciences; 2009. p. 76.

8. Akural EI, Jarvimaki V, Lansineva A, et al. Effects of combination treatment with ketoprofen 100 mg + acetaminophen 1000 mg on postoperative dental pain: a single-dose, 10-hour, randomized, double-blind, active- and placebo-controlled clinical trial. Clin Ther 2009;31(3):560–8.

9. Chang DJ, Fricke JR, Bird SR, et al. Rofecoxib versus codeine/acetaminophen in postoperative dental pain: a double-blind, randomized, placebo- and active comparator-controlled clinical trial. Clin Ther 2001;23(9):1446–55.

10. Donaldson M, Goodchild JH. Appropriate analgesic prescribing for the general dentist [review]. Gen Dent 2010;58(4):291–7 [quiz: 298–9].

11. Fricke JR Jr, Karim R, Jordan D, et al. A double-blind, single-dose comparison of the analgesic efficacy of tramadol/acetaminophen combination tablets, hydrocodone/acetaminophen combination tablets, and placebo after oral surgery. Clin Ther 2002;24(6):953–68.

12. Gatoulis SC, Voelker M, Fisher M. Assessment of the efficacy and safety profiles of aspirin and acetaminophen with codeine: results from 2 randomized, controlled trials in individuals with tension-type headache and postoperative dental pain. Clin Ther 2012;34(1):138–48.

13. Gimbel JS, Brugger A, Zhao W, et al. Efficacy and tolerability of celecoxib versus hydrocodone/acetaminophen in the treatment of pain after ambulatory orthopedic surgery in adults. Clin Ther 2001;23(2):228–41.

14. Hyllested M, Jones S, Pedersen JL, et al. Comparative effect of paracetamol, NSAIDs or their combination in postoperative pain management: a qualitative review. Br J Anaesth 2002;88:199–214.

15. Kleinert R, Lange C, Steup A, et al. Single dose analgesic efficacy of tapentadol in postsurgical dental pain: the results of a randomized, double-blind, placebo-controlled study. Anesth Analg 2008;107(6):2048–55.

16. Mehlisch DR, Aspley S, Daniels SE, et al. Comparison of the analgesic efficacy of concurrent ibuprofen and paracetamol with ibuprofen or paracetamol alone in the management of moderate to severe acute postoperative dental pain in adolescents and adults: a randomized, double-blind, placebo-controlled, parallel-group, single-dose, two-center, modified factorial study. Clin Ther 2010;32(5): 882–95.

17. Moore RA, Derry S, McQuay HJ, et al. Single dose oral analgesics for acute postoperative pain in adults [review]. Cochrane Database Syst Rev 2011;(9):CD008659.

18. Ong KS, Seymour RA. Maximizing the safety of nonsteroidal anti-inflammatory drug use for postoperative dental pain: an evidence-based approach. Anesth Prog 2003;50:62–74.

19. Tucker PW, Smith JR, Adams DF. A comparison of 2 analgesic regimens for the control of postoperative periodontal discomfort. J Periodontol 1996;67(2): 125–9.

20. Malmstrom K, Kotey P, Coughlin H, et al. A randomized, double-blind, parallel-group study comparing the analgesic effect of etoricoxib to placebo, naproxen sodium, and acetaminophen with codeine using the dental impaction pain model. Clin J Pain 2004;20(3):147–55.

21. Becker DE. Pain management: part 1: managing acute and postoperative dental pain. Anesth Prog 2010;57(2):67–78 [quiz: 79–80].

22. Ma M, Lindsell CJ, Jauch EC, et al. Effect of education and guidelines for treatment of uncomplicated dental pain on patient and provider behavior. Ann Emerg Med 2004;44(4):323–9.
23. Walker MJ, Zapata J, Lombardi AV, et al. New evidence of dental pathology in 40,000-year-old neandertals. J Dent Res 2011;90:428.
24. Runyon MS, Brennan MT, Batts JJ, et al. Efficacy of penicillin for dental pain without overt infection. Acad Emerg Med 2004;11:1268–71.
25. Roberts JR, Hedges JR. Clinical procedures in emergency medicine. 5th edition. Philadelphia: Saunders Publishing; 2009.
26. Lewis MA, Carmichael F, MacFarlane TW, et al. A randomized trial of co-amox/clav versus penicillin V in the treatment of acute dentoalveolar abscess. Br Dent J 1993; 175(5):169–74.
27. Kuriyama T, Williams DW, Yanagisawa M, et al. Antimicrobial susceptibility of 800 anaerobic isolates from patients with dentoalveolar infection to 13 oral antibiotics. Oral Microbiol Immunol 2007;22(4):285–8.
28. Matijević S, Lazić Z, Kuljić-Kapulica N, et al. Empirical antimicrobial therapy of acute dentoalveolar abscess. Vojnosanit Pregl 2009;66(7):544–50.
29. Ellison SJ. An outcome audit of three day antimicrobial prescribing for the acute dentoalveolar abscess. Br Dent J 2011;211(12):591–4.
30. Rhodus NL, Bereuter J. An evaluation of a chemical cautery agent and an anti-inflammatory ointment for the treatment of recurrent aphthous stomatitis: a pilot study. Quintessence Int 1998;29:769–73.
31. Rowland RW. Necrotizing ulcerative gingivitis. Ann Periodontol 1999;4(1):65–73 [discussion: 78].
32. Solomon LW. Chronic ulcerative stomatitis. Oral Dis 2008;14:383–9.
33. Zimmer S, Kolbe C, Kaiser G, et al. Clinical efficacy of flossing versus use of antimicrobial rinses. J Periodontol 2006;77(8):1380–5.
34. Murrell GL. Trench mouth. Otolaryngol Head Neck Surg 2010;143:599.
35. Carlson DS, Pfadt E. Vincent and Ludwig's angina: two damaging oral infections. Nursing 2011;41(2):55–8.
36. ENTemergencies: Ludwig's angina. Medscape. Available at: http://www.medscape.com/viewarticle/551650_4. Accessed February 15, 2007.
37. Rana RS, Moonis G. Head and neck infection and inflammation. Radiol Clin North Am 2011;49(1):165–82.
38. Wang LF, Tai CF, Kuo WR, et al. Predisposing factors of complicated deep neck infections: 12-year experience at a single institution. J Otolaryngol Head Neck Surg 2010;39(4):335–41.
39. Bertolai R, Acocella A, Sacco R, et al. Submandibular cellulitis (Ludwig's angina) associated to a complex odontoma erupted into the oral cavity. Case report and literature review. Minerva Stomatol 2007;56(11–12):639–47 [in English, Italian].
40. Bulut M, Balcı V, Akköse S, et al. Case report: fatal descending necrotising mediastinitis. Emerg Med J 2004;21:122–3.
41. Marioni G, Rinaldi R, Staffieri C, et al. Deep neck infection with dental origin: analysis of 85 consecutive cases (2000-2006). Acta Otolaryngol 2008;128(2): 201–6.
42. Hasan W, Leonard D, Russell J. Ludwig's angina–A controversial surgical emergency: how we do it. Int J Otolaryngol 2011;2011:231816.
43. Simon LL, Greenberg JH, Chang RS, et al. Surgical management of Ludwig's angina. ANZ J Surg 2007;77:540–3.
44. Boscolo-Rizzo P, Da Mosto MC. Submandibular space infection: a potentially lethal infection. Int J Infect Dis 2009;13(3):327–33.

45. Maestre JR, Bascones A, Sánchez P, et al. Odontogenic bacteria in periodontal disease and resistance patterns to common antibiotics used as treatment and prophylaxis in odontology in Spain. Rev Esp Quimioter 2007;20(1):61–7.
46. Kouassi YM, Janvier BB, Dufour XX, et al. Microbiology of facial cellulitis related to dental infection. Med Mal Infect 2011;41(10):540–5.
47. Fisher RG, Benjamin DK, Fisher R, et al. Facial cellulitis in childhood: a changing spectrum. South Med J 2002;95(7):672–4.

Salivary Gland Emergencies

Matthew A. Armstrong, MD, MBA[a],*, Michael A. Turturro, MD[b]

KEYWORDS

- Salivary gland • Parotitis • Sialolithiasis • Sialadenitis • Sialadenosis
- Emergency medicine

KEY POINTS

- Adult patients with acute salivary gland swelling often have bacterial infections caused by obstructive calculi in the submandibular gland and decreased salivary flow in the parotid gland, frequently due to medication side effects.
- Computed tomographic (CT) imaging is not initially required in cases of bacterial parotitis unless an abscess is suspected, the patient is septic, or the diagnosis is uncertain. Treatment of bacterial parotitis involves reversal of salivary stasis, rehydration, oral hygiene, parotid massage, sialogogues, and antibiotics.
- The most common organisms in bacterial parotitis are *Staphylococcus aureus* and oral anaerobes. However, infections are frequently polymicrobial, with mixed oral anaerobic and aerobic flora. A first-line outpatient antibiotic in bacterial parotitis is amoxicillin-clavulanate. In community-acquired cases without risk factors for methicillin-resistant *S. aureus* (MRSA) or pseudomonas, a first-line inpatient monotherapy agent is ampicillin-sulbactam.
- Pediatric patients with either unilateral or bilateral salivary gland swelling most commonly have viral infections, with mumps becoming less common. Treatment of viral parotitis is supportive with analgesics, oral hygiene, hydration, and rest. Toxic appearing patients are often treated with antibiotics in case of bacterial superinfection.
- Chronic or recurrent painful swelling may be due to obstruction, indolent infections, or autoimmune processes. A CT scan is helpful in evaluating for obstruction.
- About 80% to 90% of salivary calculi occur in the submandibular duct. Sialolithiasis is most commonly seen in middle-aged to elderly men. Attempts are made to extract distal stones from the duct. Treatment includes analgesics, regular ductal massage, sialogogues, and antibiotics in cases of overlying infection.
- Sialadenosis is noninflammatory, nonneoplastic salivary gland enlargement that is painless and usually bilateral. A wide array of disorders is responsible, including nutritional, endocrine, metabolic, autoimmune, and drug-induced. Treatment is targeted at the underlying disorder.
- Submandibular neoplasms are rare. The larger the gland, the more likely an associated mass is benign. Patients present with a progressive nonpainful, nontender mass, which may be associated with cranial neuropathies.

[a] Mike O'Callaghan Federal Hospital, Nellis Air Force Base, Las Vegas, NV, USA; [b] Department of Emergency Medicine, UPMC Mercy Hospital, 1400 Locust Street, Pittsburgh, PA 15219, USA
* Corresponding author.
E-mail address: matthew.armstrong@nellis.af.mil

Emerg Med Clin N Am 31 (2013) 481–499
http://dx.doi.org/10.1016/j.emc.2013.01.004
0733-8627/13/$ – see front matter Published by Elsevier Inc.

emed.theclinics.com

ANATOMY

Salivary production is generated principally by 3 sets of major glands: the parotid, submandibular, and sublingual glands (**Fig. 1**). In addition, there are hundreds of minor glands located in the submucosa throughout the oral cavity.

The parotid glands are the largest of the salivary glands. They wrap around the mandibular ramus on each side of the face and are roughly bordered by the following areas: anterior and inferior to the external auditory canal, inferior to the zygomatic arch, the anterior border of the masseter muscle, and along the anteromedial border of the sternocleidomastoid muscle extending to the mastoid process.[1,2] They are located mostly superficial to the masseter muscle. The facial nerve, external carotid artery, and retromandibular vein course through the parotid glands. Saliva flows away from the gland by way of Stensen duct into the oral cavity. As the duct exits the gland, it is 4 to 7 cm in diameter but narrows to approximately 0.5 mm on reaching the os.[3] The duct's orifice can be visualized directly opposite the upper second molars. In a nonpathologic state the parotid gland cannot usually be appreciated on examination; however, Stensen duct can be palpated by rolling a finger against a tensed masseter.[4]

The submandibular glands are the next largest of the salivary glands. They are located, as their name suggests, just below the mandible in the anterior portion of the submandibular triangle, which is formed by the inferior border of the mandibular body and the bellies of the digastric muscle.[2] On deep palpation normal almond-sized submandibular glands can be appreciated on each side of the neck anteroinferior to the angle of the mandible. Palpation can be optimized by having patients press

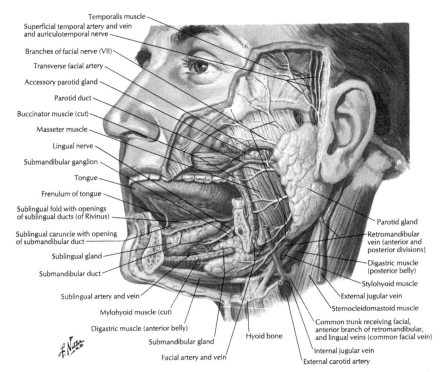

Temporalis muscle
Superficial temporal artery and vein and auriculotemporal nerve
Branches of facial nerve (VII)
Transverse facial artery
Accessory parotid gland
Parotid duct
Buccinator muscle (*cut*)
Masseter muscle
Lingual nerve
Submandibular ganglion
Tongue
Frenulum of tongue
Sublingual fold with openings of sublingual ducts (of Rivinus)
Sublingual caruncle with opening of submandibular duct
Sublingual gland
Submandibular duct
Sublingual artery and vein
Mylohyoid muscle (*cut*)
Digastric muscle (anterior belly)
Submandibular gland
Facial artery and vein
Hyoid bone
Parotid gland
Retromandibular vein (anterior and posterior divisions)
Digastric muscle (posterior belly)
Stylohyoid muscle
External jugular vein
Sternocleidomastoid muscle
Common trunk receiving facial, anterior branch of retromandibular, and lingual veins (common facial vein)
Internal jugular vein
External carotid artery

Fig. 1. The 3 major salivary glands. (Netter illustration *from* www.netterimages.com. © Elsevier Inc. All rights reserved.)

their tongue against the lower incisors, and the lobular surface can often be felt against the tightened muscle.[5] The longest of the salivary ducts, Wharton duct, drains the gland. It is 5 cm in length and 1.5 mm in diameter. The duct from each submandibular gland travels in a near vertical direction, entering the oral cavity on the floor of the mouth just lateral to the base of the frenulum of the tongue at the sublingual caruncle (**Figs. 2** and **3**). The orifice of the submandibular gland is also approximately 0.5 mm.[3]

The smallest of the major salivary gland, the sublingual glands, are located anterior to the submandibular glands, just below the mouth's floor. They lie as flat structures in a submucosal plane and normally cannot be palpated. Each gland is drained by multiple small ducts, either draining directly into the floor of the mouth or by way of the larger Wharton duct.[2] These tiny ducts empty along a ridge, the sublingual fold, running obliquely from the frenulum of the tongue (see **Figs. 2** and **3**).[6]

The minor salivary glands are plentiful and estimated to be between 600 and 1000 in the upper aerodigestive tract, being mainly concentrated in the buccal, labial, palatal, and lingual regions. They are small, 1 to 5 mm in size, and drain directly into the oral cavity through a single duct.[2]

PHYSIOLOGY

An acinus, secretory duct, and collecting duct make up the basic unit of the salivary glands. The acinus comprises a lumen surrounded by a cluster of secretory cells. Salivary gland secretions are classified as being serous, mucinous, or mixed (**Fig. 4**). Parotid glands secrete a watery serous fluid, whereas sublingual and minor glands secrete a thick mucinous fluid. The submandibular glands have mixed acini, both mucinous and serous, and secrete a semiviscous fluid.[7]

Saliva serves many functions, such as providing lubrication for swallowing, initiating digestion, modulating taste sensations, buffering pH, and defending against microorganisms. Its composition consists of water, as well as a mixture of various inorganic and organic compounds. The inorganic component is mainly electrolytes but also comprises some nitrogenous products such as urea and ammonia. The main electrolytes include sodium, potassium, calcium, magnesium, bicarbonate, and phosphate.

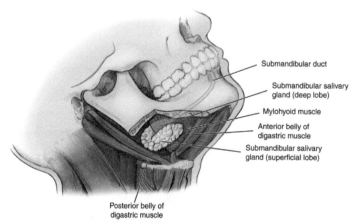

Submandibular duct

Submandibular salivary gland (deep lobe)

Mylohyoid muscle

Anterior belly of digastric muscle

Submandibular salivary gland (superficial lobe)

Posterior belly of digastric muscle

Fig. 2. Submandibular gland anatomy. The anterior and posterior bellies of the digastric muscles and the inferior border of the mandible form the submandibular triangle. (*From* Fehrenbach MJ, Herring SW. Illustrated Head and Neck Anatomy. 3 edition. St. Louis: Elsevier Saunders; 2007; with permission.)

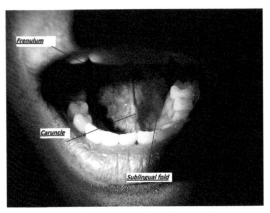

Fig. 3. Sublingual caruncle, sublingual fold, and frenulum. Wharton duct exits at the sublingual caruncle. (*Reproduced* with patient permission.)

The organic component of saliva consists of a variety of proteins such as immunoglobulins, enzymes, and mucins. These proteins play a role in antimicrobial defense, pH buffering, digestion, mineralization, lubrication, and tissue coating. Some examples include α-amylase, IgA, lactoferrin, lysozyme, peroxidase, and statherin. Mucinous glands secrete a higher concentration of antimicrobial proteins than serous glands.[7]

The composition and osmolality of saliva can change significantly depending on the salivary flow rate. Initially, the primary secretion is isotonic compared with plasma but becomes increasingly hypotonic the longer its transit through the ductal system. During this time, sodium and chloride are absorbed, whereas bicarbonate and potassium are excreted. In addition, some proteins are added to the fluid. A slower flow rate results in greater hypotonicity to the primary secretion. The composition of saliva as a whole is a combination of the secretions from each individual gland, and therefore can vary considerably depending on flow rates and relative contribution of each gland at any particular time.[7]

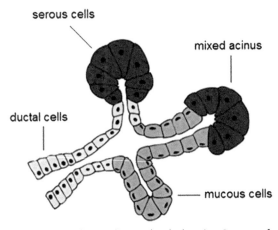

Fig. 4. Cross section of a nonrealistic salivary gland, showing 3 types of acini. (*Courtesy of* Salimetrics, LLC. Available at: www.salimetrics.com. Accessed March 3, 2012; with permission.)

The salivary system produces approximately 1 to 1.5 L of saliva daily. In the unstimulated state the submandibular gland is the largest contributor, producing 71% of saliva. The parotid and sublingual glands contribute 25% and 3% to 4%, respectively, and the minor salivary glands' contribution, relative to total daily production, is negligible. In the stimulated state, the percentage contribution of the submandibular and parotid glands is reversed, with the parotid gland being the main contributor to salivary flow.[7] With aging, salivary flow rates remain unchanged despite the degeneration of acinar cells.[2]

Salivary flow is regulated by the salivary center in the medulla. From the most potent to weakest, stimuli for increased flow are gustatory (especially acidic stimuli), the mechanical act of chewing, and olfactory. Control of flow is accomplished by way of the autonomic nervous system. Although both the sympathetic and parasympathetic components contribute to salivary flow, the parasympathetic component dominates. In general, parasympathetic stimuli results in increased salivary flow that is less viscous and less proteinaceous. The opposite is true with sympathetic stimuli.[7]

SPECIFIC DISORDERS
Sialadenitis

Inflammation can occur in any of the major salivary glands and is usually caused by infection, obstruction, or an autoimmune process. The microbiology and treatment of infections is similar for each of the salivary glands. However, retrograde nonobstructive infections are much more prevalent in the parotid glands, whereas obstructive sialadenitis, most commonly due to calculi and possibly complicated by bacterial infection, is usually observed in the submandibular glands.[8]

Parotitis
Bacterial/suppurative parotitis

Pathophysiology Suppurative parotitis is caused mainly by retrograde ascension of bacteria into Stensen duct.[8–11] Factors that decrease or inhibit salivary flow predispose to infection. These include dehydration, ductal obstruction, nerve damage, irradiation, drugs such as diuretics and those with anticholinergic activity, and chronic diseases such as diabetes mellitus, renal failure, cystic fibrosis, hypothyroidism, and Sjögren disease. Poor oral hygiene, malnutrition, tracheotomies, and periodontal disease are also risk factors.[8,12]

Dehydration can be caused by any of the usual causes such as sepsis, poor oral intake, gastrointestinal losses, medications, and blood loss. Surgery in particular is a well-established risk factor for dehydration and subsequent parotitis. In 1881, President Garfield died of parotitis following abdominal surgery.[13] Although the incidence has decreased tremendously in the era of perioperative antibiotics, parotitis still complicates between 1 in 1000 and 1 in 2000 operative procedures. This condition usually occurs within 2 weeks of the surgery, with major surgeries comprising the greatest risk.[8]

Ductal obstruction is caused by trauma, strictures, foreign bodies, sialolithiasis, and neoplasms. Lacerations of Stensen duct can lead to fistula and subsequent strictures if not properly repaired. Chronic trauma from ill-fitting dentures, prostheses, or dental irregularities can cause inflammation and swelling of the duct orifice with subsequent obstruction. Ductal obstruction from foreign bodies has been mostly reported to be due to vegetable matter, most commonly various grass seeds.[14] The incidence of this phenomenon causing clinically significant disease is unknown. As most incidences of sialolithiasis occur in the submandibular gland, salivary gland stones are a much less common cause of sialadenitis in the parotid gland compared with the submandibular gland.

Medications are a common cause of infectious sialadenitis, especially given elderly polypharmacy. Medications such as diuretics, anticholinergics, and antihistamines can cause xerostomia either by systemic dehydration or by parasympathetic inhibition. Other common classes of drugs that cause profound xerostomia include tricyclic antidepressants, monoamine oxidase inhibitors, β-blockers, barbiturates, and most neuroleptics.[15]

All major salivary glands can become infected, but the parotid gland is the most susceptible. A major reason for this is that the organic composition of parotid gland salivary excretion is less immunogenic than that of the other glands. Parotid gland saliva is serous, and unlike the mucinous saliva of the submandibular and sublingual glands, it is deficient in lysosomes, IgA antibodies, and sialic acid. In addition, mucin in mucinous saliva is composed of high-molecular-weight glycoproteins that competitively inhibit bacterial attachment to the epithelium of the salivary ducts, which provides further antimicrobial protection to the submandibular and sublingual glands.[8]

Epidemiology Although suppurative parotitis can affect persons of any age, it is predominately a disease of the middle aged and elderly. With aging, there is a higher incidence of comorbidities, polypharmacy, salivary stones, surgeries, and malnutrition, which all predispose to salivary gland infections. Most patients are between the ages of 50 and 60 years, with an equal incidence of affected men and women.[8]

Microbiology Xerostomia can lead to changes in the oral flora. Decreased oropharyngeal salivary clearance may lead to pathologic colonization with organisms such as S. aureus.[13] Not surprisingly, therefore, S. aureus is by far the most common isolated pathogen in bacterial parotitis, responsible for 50% to 90% of cases of hospitalized patients.[8] However, infections are often commonly polymicrobial; other frequently isolated organisms include viridans streptococci, Hemophilus influenza, and oral anaerobes. Gram-negative bacilli, including Enterobacteriaceae, Eikenella corrodens, Pseudomonas, and Escherichia coli are most commonly health care associated.[10,16] The oral anaerobes, including Peptostreptococcus, bacteroides species, Prevotella species, and fusobacterium, are being more frequently recognized, likely because of improved culture methods.[8] Rarer bacterial causes of parotitis include Streptococcus pneumoniae, Streptococcus pyogenes, Moraxella catarrhalis, Mycobacterium tuberculosis, and Actinomyces.[16]

Clinical presentation Patients with suppurative parotitis most commonly present with painful unilateral swelling of the cheek to the angle of the jaw. However, there is bilateral involvement in up to 25% of cases.[8] Patients may also complain of fevers, chills, malaise, trismus, and dysphagia. Patients often appear to have toxicity with high fever. They may have evidence of systemic dehydration with dry mucous membranes. Physical examination reveals a warm, erythematous, edematous, and tender parotid gland. The orifice of Stensen duct may be erythematous and pouting. Purulent material is expressed from the orifice approximately three-fourths of the time; however, drainage may not be present because of ductal obstruction or because the disease is in the early stage of development.[8] Palpation is accomplished by starting at the attachment of the earlobe and palpating in an anterior-inferior direction along the mandibular ramus. The other hand should simultaneously palpate the orifice of the Stensen duct. Not only can this result in the expression of purulent discharge, it may also reveal the presence of a salivary stone.

Diagnosis Suppurative parotitis is largely a clinical diagnosis, relying little on laboratory studies or imaging. History should review any possible risk factors for salivary gland infection. Differentiating between a viral and bacterial infectious parotitis can be a clinical enigma. In general, viral infections are bilateral, affect young patients, have prodromal symptoms, and have no purulent drainage, and patients appear to have less toxicity. Although systemic symptoms follow the development of a symptomatic gland in suppurative parotitis, the order is usually reversed in viral parotitis.

Although laboratory studies and imaging are not necessary for a diagnosis, these often reveal a leukocytosis with neutrophilia. In contrast to mumps, the serum amylase level is typically normal in suppurative parotitis.[8]

If pus is expressed from Stensen duct, it should be sent for Gram staining and culture. Specimens should be cultured for aerobic and anaerobic bacteria, fungi, and mycobacteria. The primary utility of these cultures is for susceptibility testing to determine the need to adjust antimicrobial therapy in the individual patient. These results, however, should ultimately be interpreted with caution given the possibility of intraoral flora contamination. Percutaneous aspiration of the involved gland is the ideal test but is usually reserved for ear, nose and throat (ENT) specialists.

Imaging is not usually necessary on initial presentation. However, if there is no improvement after 48 hours, imaging is recommended to evaluate for abscess or an obstructive process such as calculus.[8] Imaging is also reasonable when the patient appears to have toxicity or sepsis, if there is suspicion for abscess, or if the diagnosis is uncertain. Possible imaging options include CT scan, magnetic resonance (MR) sialography, or ultrasonography (US). A maxillofacial CT with intravenous (IV) contrast is the most sensitive and commonly used tool for detecting an abscess.[16] Fine cuts must be specified to better identify possible calculi. US is becoming a more frequently used modality, especially in patients with contraindications to IV contrast. US can detect greater than 90% of stones 2 mm or more.[3] MR sialography does not require the injection of intraductal dye. It can assess the ductal architecture and is possibly superior to US in stone detection but is limited by time requirements and is not currently widely used.

Differential diagnosis Bacterial parotitis must be differentiated from other causes of facial swelling and pain (**Tables 1** and **2**). In cases in which an exudative drainage can be expressed from Stensen duct, the diagnosis is straight forward. However, exudative drainage is not always present, which can make the diagnosis more challenging. Viral parotitis typically presents after a few days of systemic prodromal symptoms before symptomatic gland involvement. Patients tend to be young and appear to have less toxicity. In contrast to the unilateral involvement of suppurative parotitis, viral parotitis usually produces bilateral pain and swelling, usually without overlying warmth and erythema. Elevation of serum amylase level is more common than in suppurative parotitis. Viral infections due to mumps can have classic concurrent complications including orchitis or aseptic meningitis. Pain associated with an acute salivary stone, whether or not associated with infection, begins acutely, is unilateral, and is periprandial. Patients are uncomfortable but appear well. Often a stone can be palpated along Stensen duct. In chronic recurrent parotitis, a stone or other obstruction can cause recurrent episodes of swelling and pain that is periprandial. Nonneoplastic salivary gland swelling, sialadenosis, is usually bilateral, painless, and persistent. There may be stigmata of autoimmune disease. Neoplastic swelling is unilateral, painless, with progressive nodular growth. There may be associated facial nerve palsy.

Other nonsalivary gland causes of swelling include lymphangitis, lymphoma, otitis externa, buccal space abscess, masseteric space abscess, canine space abscess, parapharyngeal abscess, extension of mastoiditis into sternocleidomastoid (Bezold abscess), odontogenic infections, Ludwig angina, infected branchial cleft, or sebaceous cysts.

Table 1
Differential diagnosis of parotid gland swelling and/or pain

Parotid Gland Related	Non–Parotid Gland Related
Acute	Lymphadenopathy
Bacterial parotitis	Lymphadenitis
Viral parotitis	Lymphoma
Sialolithiasis	Otitis externa
Pneumoparotitis	Buccal space abscess
Persistent	Masseteric space abscess
Tuberculosis	Canine space abscess
Cat-scratch disease	Parapharyngeal abscess
Sjögren disease	Bezold abscess
Toxoplasmosis	Odontogenic infections
Actinomycosis	Ludwig angina
Fungal	Infected branchial cleft cyst
Sarcoidosis/Heerfordt syndrome	Infected sebaceous cyst
Anorexia nervosa	
Bulimia	
Malnutrition	
Vitamin deficiency	
Malabsorption	
Hypothyroidism	
Diabetes mellitus	
Acromegaly	
Gonadal hypofunction	
Obesity	
Cirrhosis	
Pregnancy	
Iodine-containing contrast	
Heavy metals	
Certain medications	
Alcoholism	
Recurrent	
Sialolithiasis	
Recurrent parotitis of childhood	
Pneumoparotitis	
Progressive	
Neoplasm	

Treatment Management of suppurative parotitis, besides any necessary emergency stabilization, includes reversal of salivary stasis, rehydration, oral hygiene, parotid massage, sialogogues, and antibiotics. All pharmacologic agents that result in salivary stasis should be discontinued whenever possible. Analgesics and local heat application can provide symptomatic relief. Parotid massage should be performed regularly by the patients if possible, starting from the gland and working along the course of the duct. Although temporarily painful, this maneuver helps relieve the pressure and associated pain. Potent sialogogues such as lemon drops or orange juice should be regularly used to stimulate salivary flow. Good oral hygiene of regular brushing and flossing should be recommended.

Antibiotics are the mainstay of therapy, and their administration should be timely. Appropriate empiric antibiotic regimens should include coverage for *S. aureus* as well as oral polymicrobial aerobic and anaerobic infections. A high percentage of infections caused by β-lactamase–producing bacteria (75% in one study) necessitate treatment with an antistaphylococcal penicillin, a combination β-lactamase inhibitor,

Table 2
Causes of parotid gland swelling and/or pain

Type	Onset	Symmetry	Pain	General Appearance	Fever	Stensen Duct	Palpation	Other Clues
Suppurative parotitis	Acute	Unilateral (75%)	+	Toxic	+	Pus	Tender, erythema and warmth	Middle aged/elderly, medications, dehydration
Viral parotitis	Systemic prodrome	Bilateral (75%)	+	Mild to moderately ill	±	Inflamed orifice	Tender, no erythema or warmth	Children, possible aseptic meningitis or orchitis if mumps
Obstructive (without infection)	Periprandial	Unilateral	±	Well	-	Possible stone	Tender	Adults, may resolve between meals
Chronic parotitis	Persistent or recurrent	Varies	±	Well	-	Normal	Nontender	Often obstruction, possible associated rheumatoid disease
Neoplastic	Progressive	Unilateral	-	Well	-	Normal	Often discrete nodule	Possible facial palsy
Sialadenosis	Persistent	Bilateral	-	Well	-	Normal	Nontender	Often malnutrition, endocrine, or medications
Pneumoparotitis	Acute	Varies	-	Well	-	Frothy discharge	Crepitus	Glassblower, wind instrumentalists, or maladaptive behavior

or a first-generation cephalosporin.[17] Potential first-line parental regimens for inpatient management include nafcillin or cefazolin combined with clindamycin or metronidazole (Flagyl).[16] Another option is monotherapy with ampicillin-sulbactam (Unasyn).[15] Patients allergic to penicillin can be treated with a macrolide such as azithromycin plus metronidazole. In patients with risk factors for MRSA, vancomycin or linezolid should be substituted for nafcillin or added to ampicillin-sulbactam. Risk factors for MRSA include recent hospitalization, recent antibiotic therapy, hemodialysis, diabetes mellitus, or residence in a long-term-care facility.[16] In addition, patients who are immunocompromised or recently hospitalized or come from a long-term-care facility should be treated with coverage for Enterobacteriaceae and *Pseudomonas aeruginosa*. Options for such patients are vancomycin or linezolid plus piperacillin-tazobactom (Zosyn), imipenem, meropenem, or cefepime combined with metronidazole. Antibiotic therapy may need to be modified later in the inpatient setting based on culture results. In cases of abscess formation, surgical drainage by ENT specialists is necessary.

Due to potentially devastating complications including abscess formation, sepsis, mandibular osteomyelitis, internal jugular vein thrombophlebitis, respiratory obstruction and death, admission is typically recommended for most patients with suppurative parotitis.[10–12,16] However, complications are rare, and outpatient management can be considered in patients who are well-appearing with no systemic involvement, have no significant comorbidities, and who are able to tolerate oral intake with close outpatient follow-up arranged.[9,15] A first-line oral outpatient antibiotic is amoxicillin-clavulanate (Augmentin). Patients allergic to penicillin can be treated with a macrolide plus metronidazole. Monotherapy with clindamycin should also be adequate for the vast majority of patients in community-acquired cases to cover both *S. aureus* and anaerobes. It would not, however, provide any coverage for the minority of patients requiring gram-negative coverage, including for *H. influenza* or *M. catarrhalis*. ENT follow-up should be established and should generally occur within the first few days following emergency department (ED) discharge.

Complications The mortality of suppurative parotitis has improved dramatically in the era of antibiotics but is still reported to be 20% to 40%.[4] Potential complications are rare but can be serious. These include abscess formation and extension into deep spaces of the neck, face, and mediastinum; sepsis; osteomyelitis of the mandible; septic thrombophlebitis of the jugular vein (Lemierre syndrome); respiratory obstruction; rupture through the floor of the external auditory canal; and spontaneous drainage through the face. Facial nerve palsy can also occur but is rare and more commonly associated with parotid malignancy. Not specific to parotitis, strictures can occur in any involved salivary duct after an episode of infectious sialadenitis, potentially resulting in recurrent infections.[18]

Viral parotitis
Pathophysiology Bacterial parotitis is most commonly caused by retrograde ductal bacterial seeding, whereas viral infections are most commonly spread hematogenously.[8] However, retrograde infections do occur, as is the case of mumps, the classic viral parotitis.[8,15] In mumps, the paramyxovirus virus is disseminated by airborne droplets from salivary, nasal, and urinary secretions. These droplets enter the upper respiratory tract and directly invade the upper respiratory tract epithelium as well as the parotid duct and gland. There is an incubation period of 2 to 3 weeks while the virus multiplies before the virus spreads hematogenously and patients become symptomatic.[8]

Epidemiology Viral parotitis occurs more commonly in young patients than suppurative parotitis. In mumps, in particular, 85% of cases occur in children younger than

15 years.[8] The current incidence of viral parotitis is unknown. However, since the advent of a live attenuated mumps vaccine in 1967, the incidence of mumps has dropped dramatically in the United States from 152,209 cases in 1968 to only 370 cases in 2011.[19]

Virology Classically, mumps parotitis has been nearly synonymous with nonsuppurative viral parotitis. It has been reported to be by far the most common cause of viral parotitis, even in the postvaccine era.[8] However, this assertion is principally based on data from the 1960s.[20] Later evidence suggests that mumps may not be as common a cause of parotitis as it once was. During an outbreak of mumps in Nova Scotia in 2007, only 14% of the 2082 cases that were reported to be mumps were later serologically confirmed, which may have been due to low sensitivity of the confirmatory assays. However, physician inexperience in recognizing mumps infection versus other causes of acute parotitis may have contributed to the low positivity rate reported.[21] In Finland, of 601 cases clinically suspected to be mumps during the period 1983 to 1998, only 17 (2%) patients actually had a confirmed mumps virus infection.[22] In this study, an alternative viral cause could only be confirmed in 14% of the cases. The remaining 86% of patients may have had a noninfectious cause of parotitis, a viral infection that was not detected, insensitive studies, or a non parotid gland related cause of their symptoms. In those patients with positive viral serologic test results, the most common causes of viral parotitis were Epstein-Barr, followed by parainfluenza, human herpesvirus 6, adenovirus, enterovirus, and parvovirus.

Other viruses that can cause parotitis include influenza, coxsackie, enteric cytopathic human orphan virus, cytomegalovirus, lymphocytic choriomeningitic virus, and human immunodeficiency virus.[8,15] These cases of viral parotitis are isolated, sporadic, and often erroneously labeled as mumps.[23]

Clinical presentation Before salivary gland swelling, patients typically experience 3 to 5 days of nonspecific prodromal symptoms, which may include fever, malaise, headache, myalgias, arthralgias, and anorexia. Depending on the virus, the patient may also have concurrent upper respiratory symptoms. Patients then develop pain and swelling, usually of the parotid gland, but any of the salivary glands may be involved. In 75% of cases the involvement is bilateral.[8] However, patients may initially have unilateral involvement, then develop bilateral pain and swelling during the next few days. Patients may have associated earache, fever, trismus, and dysphagia.

Physical examination may reveal fever with a mildly to moderately ill general appearance. Patients have swelling and tenderness over the involved glands. However, erythema and warmth should not be present over the face.[9] The opening to Stensen duct may appear inflamed, but purulent drainage should not be present with ductal massage. In the case of mumps, patients may have evidence of orchitis, oophoritis, mastitis, pancreatitis, hearing loss, encephalitis, or aseptic meningitis.

Diagnosis Similar to suppurative parotitis, viral parotitis is a clinical diagnosis. If laboratory studies are obtained, they may reveal an elevated serum amylase level and leukocytopenia with a relative lymphocytosis.[9] However, a white blood cell (WBC) count, as in most other disease processes, is neither sensitive nor specific. The WBC count may be low, normal, or elevated in viral parotitis. For epidemiologic purposes, if mumps is suspected, especially in the unimmunized and those with an epidemiologic link, serology and buccal swabs should be obtained. Mumps testing should be performed both of the buccal mucosa around Stensen duct and of the serum.[24] Either enzyme immunoassays or immunofluorescence assays can be ordered to detect IgM and IgG paramyxovirus antibodies. The presence of IgM signifies a primary infection, whereas the isolated presence of IgG represents prior exposure or vaccination. Repeat assays should be obtained during the convalescent phase in 2 weeks. A 4-fold increase or conversion of IgG at that time is diagnostic of an acute infection with the mumps virus.[8] Buccal swabs should also be sent for viral culture and reverse transcriptase polymerase chain reaction (RT-PCR) to detect the RNA of paramyxovirus. RT-PCR is highly sensitive and specific as an inherent test.[25] However, the sensitivity can vary substantially in clinical practice based on the timing of collection and the quality of the sample.[24] In addition, IgM serologic testing is often negative in previously immunized patients, as these patients predominately mount a secondary immune response. During one outbreak in 2007 in Nova Scotia, the sensitivity for RT-PCR and IgM serology was 79% and 25%, respectively.[21] Therefore, negative testing does not necessarily rule out an active mumps infection, especially in partially immunized individuals.

Prevention The measles, mumps, and rubella vaccination is recommended by the Center for Disease Control (CDC) to be administered as 2 doses, the first between 12 and 15 months of age and the second between the ages of 4 and 6 years. This vaccination confers immunity 62% to 91% of the time in patients who have received 1 dose and 76% to 95% in those who have received both.[26]

Differential diagnosis The differential diagnosis for viral parotitis is similar to that of bacterial parotitis (see Differential Diagnosis in section Bacterial/Suppurative Parotitis).

Treatment Treatment of viral parotitis is supportive and includes hydration, oral hygiene, and rest. Antipyretics, antiinflammatories, and/or analgesics are beneficial. Although not part of the treatment of viral infections, antibiotics are often prescribed by practitioners when the diagnosis is uncertain or patients appear to have toxicity.[23] Certain states require that probable or confirmed cases of mumps be reported to the state health department. Patients should be given follow-up with their primary care physician for repeat serologic testing. Patients with a presumptive diagnosis of viral parotitis should be instructed regarding potential complications of mumps. They should practice good hand hygiene and remain isolated at home for 5 days from the onset of parotitis symptoms.[27] Fever abatement usually precedes the resolution of parotid swelling, which typically takes 5 to 10 days.[28]

Complications Mumps is usually benign, and complications are rare. However, the disease is more severe in adults. Potential complications include orchitis in men, oophoritis in women, mastitis, pancreatitis, aseptic meningitis, sensorineural hearing loss, myocarditis, polyarthritis, hemolytic anemia, and thrombocytopenia.[9] Mumps infection in the first trimester of pregnancy has been associated with an increased rate of spontaneous abortion but is not associated with congenital malformations.[23] All viral infections can be complicated by a superimposed bacterial infection due to ductal inflammation and obstruction.

Chronic parotitis Chronic sialadenitis is characterized clinically as recurrent or persistent painful swelling of the salivary glands that most commonly involves the parotid glands.[8] Several different, often contradictory, classification systems have been proposed for this entity.[29] For their purposes, the authors include any process that causes chronic parotid inflammation. This condition can have multiple causes, including obstructive, infectious, and autoimmune mediated. However, the final common pathway is progressive acinar destruction with fibrous replacement and sialectasis.

A simplified approach involves determining whether the cause is obstructive or not. A high-resolution noncontrast CT scan with requested fine cuts through the gland has a high sensitivity for detecting stones, an extrinsically compressing tumor, or foreign body.[8] A sialogram can detect any strictures or congenital dilatation but is not usually readily obtainable from the ED and should not be performed if suppurative parotitis is suspected. These obstructions can predispose patients to recurrent or persistent episodes of inflammation and infection. A low-grade chronic infection or acute episodes of suppurative parotitis may result.

Nonobstructive infectious causes include cat-scratch disease, toxoplasmosis, mycobacterial disease, actinomycosis, and fungal infections.[30] Noninfectious causes include Sjögren disease; sarcoidosis; Heerfordt syndrome, which is a distinct presentation of sarcoidosis manifested as uveoparotitis, fever, and often cranial nerve VII palsy.[23]

Patients with an acute episode of suppurative parotitis should be treated accordingly. Otherwise, most causes of chronic symptoms do not require emergent intervention and can be treated supportively with hydration and analgesics. Based on clinical suspicion, the patient should be directed to appropriate follow-up, which may include otorhinolaryngology, infectious disease, and/or rheumatology for definitive diagnosis and treatment. Based on the suspected underlying cause and possibly in counsel with the specialist, diagnostic studies including rheumatoid serologic testing and ductal secretion cultures may be obtained.

Recurrent parotitis of childhood   Although rare, recurrent parotitis of childhood (RPC) is the second most common inflammatory cause of parotitis in children, with viral parotitis being the most common.[31] The cause of this disorder is unknown but is thought to be secondary to congenital sialectasis predisposing to recurrent retrograde bacterial seeding of the ductal system.[8,31] The age of onset is between 8 months and 16 years, with a peak incidence between 3 and 6 years. Episodes usually last for a few days and occur 6 to 8 times per year. Boys are affected more commonly than girls.[8]

Patients present with recurrent episodes of unilateral or bilateral (44% of cases) parotid gland pain and swelling.[8] Often, patients have associated systemic symptoms of fever and malaise. Typically, no purulent drainage can be expressed from Stensen duct, helping to distinguish RPC from suppurative parotitis.

In the past, diagnosis was confirmed by conventional sialogram, which revealed formation of punctate or globular sialectasis scattered throughout the gland as demonstrated by multiple round pools of contrast medium about 2 to 3 mm in size.[8] However, ultrasound imaging is quickly becoming the initial test of choice, as it is noninvasive and equally as sensitive as a conventional siolagram.[32] Findings on ultrasound imaging of RPC include multiple hypoechoic nodules in the gland suggestive of sialectasis. Ultrasound imaging can also be helpful in detecting any stones, masses, or abscesses.

Treatment of RPC is controversial. As the average amount of delay in diagnosis is more than 1 year, the patient may have already had an extensive work-up and received multiple antibiotic courses. If not performed previously, testing for mumps should be considered and bacterial cultures obtained. Although once the diagnosis is established antibiotics are not recommended, conservative treatment with antibiotics is recommended until suppurative parotitis is excluded.[23,32] The most commonly isolated organisms from patients with RPC are S. aureus and Streptococcus viridans. Intravenous antibiotics, similar to those in suppurative parotitis, should be initiated in patients who appear to have toxicity, who are unable to tolerate oral intake, or in whom close otorhinolaryngologic follow-up cannot be ensured. Empiric outpatient antibiotic therapy should consist of a penicillinase-resistant antistaphylococcal antibiotic, such as amoxicillin-clavulanate. Additional treatment includes hydration, oral hygiene, sialogogues, warm compresses, and analgesics.

Pneumoparotitis   Pneumoparotitis is also known as wind parotitis and surgical or anesthesia mumps, and air within the ducts and parenchyma of the parotid gland causes swelling. The mechanism consists of increased intraoral pressure, causing insufflation of Stensen duct, which may be associated with overlying inflammation. It is an occupational hazard for glassblowers and wind instrumentalists, including trumpet and windpipe players. Other causes include positive pressure ventilation, dental instrumentation, voluntary cough suppression, and maladaptive behavior in children.[33]

Patients may present with painless, unilateral or bilateral, and nontender swelling of the parotid gland with a history consistent with injury. However, tenderness, warmth, and overlying may be present if associated with infectious parotitis. Crepitus may be appreciated on palpation, and frothy air-filled saliva may be expressed from Stensen duct. If CT imaging is obtained because of suspicion for other causes of swelling, it reveals air in the parotid duct and gland. Potential complications include dissection of air causing subcutaneous emphysema with airway compromise, pneumomediastinum, or pneumothorax. Repetitive injury may result in sialectasis, causing salivary stasis and the risk of recurrent bacterial infection. Treatment of a single episode requires only behavior adaptation, reassurance, and prophylactic antistaphylococcal penicillinase-resistant antibiotics such as amoxicillin-clavulanate. Recurrent episodes, especially when sialectasis is suspected or seen on imaging, require ENT follow-up and may eventually require surgical intervention.[33] Superimposed cases of bacterial parotitis require appropriate antibiotic treatment, sialogogues, hydration, massage, warm compresses, and disposition as previously described.

Sialadenitis of the submandibular and sublingual glands
All the processes that cause parotitis can also occur in the other salivary glands but are less common. The only exception to this is sialadenitis caused by stones, with the vast majority of cases of sialolithiasis occurring in the submandibular glands. When infectious sialadenitis does occur, often preceded by obstruction, the microbiology and treatment are the same as in the parotid gland. Radiographs and CT imaging are of higher yield than in the parotid gland because of a greater likelihood of a radiopaque obstructing stone. Ludwig angina must be ruled out when infection is suspected. Treatment of sialadenitis is targeted at the cause of inflammation whether infectious, obstructive, or autoimmune as directed throughout this article.

Sialolithiasis

Pathophysiology
Salivary stones are formed when an organic matrix of glycoproteins and mucopolysaccharide gels combines with calcium carbonate and calcium phosphate in a stagnant duct.[8] Although the exact cause of this process remains unclear, most agree that salivary stasis and ductal inflammation contribute. Some of the same causes of salivary stasis that predispose to infectious sialadenitis, including dehydration, medications, and malnutrition, also contribute to salivary gland stone formation.[3] In fact, these 2 processes, sialolithiasis and infectious sialadenitis, likely are often interconnected with one process predisposing to and often preceding the other.[8,34]

Of all salivary stones found in Wharton duct, 80% to 90% are from the submandibular gland, with the vast majority of the remaining ones found in Stensen duct.[35] This predilection for the submandibular gland is likely due in part to the fact that Wharton duct is longer, wider, and nearly vertically angulated against gravity, all of which contribute to salivary stasis. In addition, the semimucous secretion of the submandibular gland is more viscous compared with the serous secretion of the parotid gland.[8,35]

Epidemiology
Sialolithiasis can occur in patients of any age but most frequently occurs in patients in their fifth to eighth decade of life and is much more commonly seen in men than women.[8]

Clinical presentation

Patients with an acute salivary stone present after a sudden onset of colicky peripran-dial pain associated with salivary gland swelling. The pain and swelling may be recur-rent, associated occasionally with meals. The involved gland is tender, but there should not be any expressible ductal purulent drainage or overlying erythema or warmth unless there is concurrent infection. On bimanual palpation, a stone can often be felt along the course of the involved gland's duct.[35]

Diagnosis

In the absence of a palpable stone, the diagnosis of sialolithiasis can often be chal-lenging, especially in the differentiation from infectious sialadenitis, which can, on occasion, be simultaneously present. Isolated sialolithiasis is predominately unilateral with no associated purulent drainage, no overlying erythema, and no systemic symp-toms such as fever. A key historical feature is the periprandial sudden onset.

Sialolithiasis is confirmed radiographically. Plain film radiography is inexpensive and rapid, results in minimal radiation exposure, and may confirm the diagnosis. It is most useful in submandibular stones where 90% of the stones are radiopaque, as opposed to only 20% to 40% of parotid gland stones.[3,8,35] Intraoral radiography, performed at 90° from the floor of the mouth, is best at detecting radiopaque stones in Wharton duct. However, other calcifications such as phleboliths, calcified cervical lymphade-nopathy, and arterial atherosclerosis of the lingual artery can make interpretation more difficult.[34] Noncontrasted CT imaging with fine cuts provide excellent sensitivity and is commonly used but is associated with increased radiation exposure. Ultra-sound imaging has proved to be valuable, when available, because of its ability to detect 90% of stones greater than 2 mm.[3] As in CT, ultrasound imaging can reveal additional data such as the presence of an abscess or mass.

Treatment

Patients with evidence of overlying suppurative sialadenitis should be treated with antibiotics as previously described. Attempts at removing palpable stones located near the orifices of the ducts may be successful by digitally "milking" the stones out. If the practitioner is comfortable with the procedure and the associated anatomy, attempts can be made to dilate or incise the orifice of Wharton duct to aid in extraction. A 00 lacrimal probe or a blunt, rigid, slightly beveled cannula is used for the dilatation. To perform the surgical incision of the duct papilla, local anesthesia is first obtained by submucosal injection of the papilla or a lingual block is performed. One blade of straight iris scissors is placed in the orifice while a small pair of toothed forceps provides gentle traction. The orifice and up to approximately 1.25 cm of Wharton duct is incised. Gentle massage can help advance the stone into the enlarged lumen. No suturing of the marsupialized orifice and proximal duct is necessary. Potential complications of this procedure include trauma to the lingual nerve (which is just deep to the submandibular duct), the sublingual veins, and the sublingual gland (which are located medially and laterally, respectively, to the Wharton duct's orifice).[34] There-fore, this procedure should be performed only by a physician with previous experience performing duct papillary incision.

Regardless of the success in extraction, patients should be given otorhinolaryngo-logic or oral surgery follow-up and be treated with analgesics, regular ductal massage by the patient, and sialogogues, such as lemon drops or orange juice. If conservative treatment fails, further management may include surgical intervention, whether by an intraoral or cervical approach; lithotripsy; or sialoendoscopy using a rigid endoscope with a combination of baskets, graspers, and intracorporeal lithotripsy.[3]

Sialadenosis

Sialadenosis is noninflammatory, nonneoplastic salivary gland enlargement. Histology reveals acinar hypertrophy without an inflammatory infiltrate.[36] Sialadenosis can result from a large number of conditions, and the pathophysiology is not well understood. Causes of sialadenosis include anorexia nervosa; bulimia; malnutrition with vitamin deficiency, including beriberi and pellagra; diabetes; malabsorption; hypothyroidism; acromegaly; gonadal hypofunction; obesity; alcoholic cirrhosis; alcoholism; pregnancy; chronic pancreatitis; iodine-containing contrast media; heavy metals; and certain drugs such as phenylbutazone, thiouracil, isoproterenol; and phenothiazines such as prochlorperazine.[15,36]

Typically, this condition involves the parotid glands. Patients present with painless swelling that is often bilateral, but it can also be unilateral. On examination, the patient does not appear to have toxicity, and the involved glands are nontender with no overlying erythema or warmth. There is no purulent drainage from the involved gland's duct. Emergency intervention is usually not required in sialadenosis. Treatment generally consists of addressing the underlying cause. Definitive outpatient care is the rule. Patients should be discharged with appropriate follow-up based on the suspected underlying cause.[15]

Neoplasms

Only 3% to 4% of all head and neck tumors occur in the salivary glands. Around 80% of salivary gland neoplasms occur in the parotid gland, with the vast majority of the remainder occurring in the submandibular and minor glands.[37] As a general rule, the larger the size of the gland, the higher the odds of a mass being benign.[3] In one large review of 2410 patients, 14% of sublingual, 63% of submandibular, and 85% of parotid neoplasms were benign. Minor salivary gland tumors made up 14% of the neoplasms, with 46% of those being malignant.[38] The incidence of malignancy increases with age and peaks between the ages of 65 and 74 years. However, although the occurrence of neoplasms is low in children, a high percentage of salivary gland masses are malignant.[8]

Patients present with chronic, progressive, painless swelling of the involved salivary gland. Minor gland neoplasms may cause painless masses or ulcerations in the oral mucosa. Tumors may present at advanced stages with intracranial extension and cranial nerve neuropathies. If present in the nasal cavity or maxillary sinus, they may lead to chronic congestion, nasal obstruction, or sinusitis.[39] Laryngeal minor salivary gland tumors may cause airway obstruction, dysphagia, or hoarseness. If a parotid tumor extends into the infratemporal fossa, there may be associated trismus. Extrinsic compression of salivary ducts may result in pain, swelling, and overlying infection. As a rule, facial nerve paralysis indicates that the swelling is due to a neoplastic process. Physical examination may reveal a discrete, nontender mass. Evidence of cranial nerve involvement includes trismus, hoarseness, asymmetric palatal elevation, decreased gag reflex, and facial nerve palsy. Regional lymphadenopathy may be present.

Uncomplicated cases with small lesions simply require urgent outpatient specialist follow-up for possible ultrasonography and fine-needle aspiration. Patients with cranial nerve palsies, concern for invasion, or overlying infection likely merit advanced imaging and admission with ENT consultation. MRI and CT imaging with IV contrast are able to assess for extension and complications, with CT being more expeditious.

Cysts and Mucoceles

Mucoceles and mucous retention cysts are common oral lesions. Mucous retention cysts form when the tiny ducts of a minor salivary gland become obstructed, causing

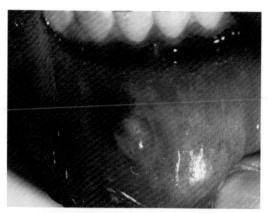

Fig. 5. A mucocele. (*Courtesy of* Logical Images, Inc. All rights reserved; with permission.)

mucin-filled cysts. Mucoceles are clinically similar appearing to retention cysts but are much more common (**Fig. 5**). Histologically, however, mucoceles are pseudocysts not containing an epithelial lining and form when mucin from damaged or obstructed ducts extravasates into the surrounding soft tissues. These fluid-filled lesions occur predominately in children and young adults. They occur most commonly in the lower lip when trauma, frequently from lip biting, causes disruption of the duct. They can vary in size and may occur as translucent pinkish or blue soft papules or nodules. They may spontaneously rupture and resolve. Drainage is not recommended in the acute setting. The lesions may ultimately require excision or marsupialization by an appropriate specialist.[40]

Ranulas are mucoceles specifically of the sublingual gland (**Fig. 6**). Rarely, they extend into the neck through the myolohyoid muscle, causing swelling, and are then described as "plunging." Complete excision, often with the associated sublingual gland, is the preferred treatment.[41]

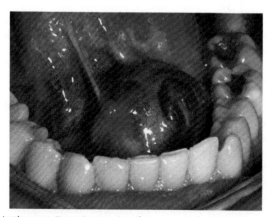

Fig. 6. From the Latin root "rana" meaning frog, a ranula appears as a blue translucent swelling in the floor of the mouth reminiscent of the underbelly of a frog. (*Courtesy of* Logical Images, Inc. All rights reserved; with permission.)

REFERENCES

1. Flatau AT, Mills PR. Anatomy and physiology. In: Norman JE, McGurk M, editors. Color atlas and text of the salivary glands: diseases, disorders, and surgery. London: Mosby-Wolfe; 1995. p. 13.
2. Holsinger CF, Bui DT. Anatomy, function, and evaluation of the salivary glands. In: Myers EN, Ferris RL, editors. Salivary gland disorders. Berlin: Springer; 2007. p. 2–9.
3. Fazio S, Emerick K. Salivary gland stones. In: Basow D, editor. UpToDate. Waltham (MA): UpToDate; 2012. Accessed December 17, 2011.
4. McAnally T. Parotitis: clinical presentations and management. Postgrad Med 1982;71(2):87–93.
5. Bickley LS, Szilagyi PG. The head and neck. In: Bickley LS, editor. Bates' guide to physical examination and history taking. 8th edition. Philadelphia: Lippincott Williams & Wilkins; 2003. p. 115.
6. O'Rahilly R, Muller F, Carpenter S, et al. Basic human anatomy: a regional study of human structure. Chapter 51: The mouth, tongue, and teeth. 2008. Available at: http://www.dartmouth.edu/~humananatomy/part_8/chapter_51.html. Accessed January 27, 2012.
7. Elluru RG. Physiology of the salivary glands. In: Flint PW, editor. Cummings otolaryngology head & neck surgery, vol. 2, 5th edition. Philadelphia: Elsevier Mosby; 2010. p. 1133–42.
8. Rogers J, McCaffrey TV. Inflammatory disorders of the salivary glands. In: Flint PW, editor. Cummings otolaryngology head & neck surgery, vol. 2, 5th edition. Philadelphia: Elsevier Mosby; 2010. p. 1151–61.
9. McQuone SJ. Acute viral and bacterial infections of the salivary glands. Otolaryngol Clin North Am 1999;32(5):793–811.
10. Brook I. Acute bacterial suppurative parotitis: microbiology and management. J Craniofac Surg 2003;14(1):37–40.
11. Brook I. Diagnosis and management of parotitis. Arch Otolaryngol Head Neck Surg 1992;118(5):469–71.
12. Al-Dajani N, Wootton SH. Cervical lymphadenitis, suppurative parotitis, thyroiditis, and infected cysts. Infect Dis Clin North Am 2007;21(2):523–41, viii.
13. Cawson RA, Eveson JW, Gleeson MJ. Sialadenitis. In: Cawson RA, Eveson JW, Gleeson MJ, editors. Pathology and surgery of the salivary glands. Oxford: ISIS Medical; 1997. p. 1–34.
14. Bailey BJ. Salivary glands-trauma. In: Cummings CW, Fredrickson JM, et al, editors. Otolaryngology head and neck surgery. 3rd edition. St. Louis: Mosby; 1998. p. 302–17.
15. Tintinalli J, Kelen G, Stapczynski J. Face and jaw emergencies. In: Tintinalli J, editor. Emergency medicine: a comprehensive study guide. 6th edition. New York: McGraw-Hill; 2004. p. 752–5.
16. Chow A. Suppurative parotitis in adults. In: Basow D, editor. UpToDate. Waltham (MA): UpToDate; 2012. Accessed December 17, 2011.
17. Brook I, Frazier EH, Thompson DH. Aerobic and anaerobic microbiology of acute suppurative parotitis. Laryngoscope 1991;101(2):170–2.
18. Ngu RK, Brown JE, Whaites EJ, et al. Salivary duct strictures: nature and incidence in benign salivary obstruction. Dentomaxillofac Radiol 2007;36(2):63–7.
19. Center for Disease Control. NNDSS tables. Provisional cases of selected notifiable diseases, United States. Available at: http://wonder.cdc.gov/mmwr/mmwr_reps.asp?mmwr_year=2011&mmwr_week=52&mmwr_table=2G. Accessed February 28, 2012.

20. Cherry JD, Jahn CL. Exanthem and dnanthem associated with mumps virus infection. Arch Environ Health 1966;12(4):518–21.
21. Hatchette TF, Mahony JB, Chong S, et al. Difficulty with mumps diagnosis: what is the contribution of mumps mimickers? J Clin Virol 2009;46(4):381–3.
22. Davidkin I, Jokinen S, Paananen A, et al. Etiology of mumps-like illnesses in children and adolescents vaccinated for measles, mumps, and rubella. J Infect Dis 2005;191(5):719–23.
23. Marchal F, Bradley PJ. Management of infections of the salivary glands. In: Myers EN, Ferris RL, editors. Salivary gland disorders. Berlin: Springer; 2007. p. 2–9.
24. Center for Disease Control. Questions and Answers about Lab Testing. Available at: http://www.cdc.gov/mumps/lab/qa-lab-test-infect.html. Accessed February 28, 2012.
25. Boddicker JD, Rota PA, Kreman T, et al. Real-time reverse transcription-PCR assay for detection of mumps virus RNA in clinical specimens. J Clin Microbiol 2007;45(9):2902–8.
26. Center for Disease Control. Mumps Testing. Available at: http://www.cdc.gov/mumps/vaccination.html. Accessed February 28, 2012.
27. Center for Disease Control. Patient isolation. Available at: http://www.cdc.gov/mumps/prev-control-settings/patient-isolation.html. Accessed February 28, 2012.
28. Albrecht MA. Epidemiology, clinical manifestations, diagnosis, and management of mumps. In: Basow D, editor. UpToDate. Waltham (MA): UpToDate; 2012. Accessed December 17, 2011.
29. Wang S, Marchal F, Zou Z, et al. Classification and management of chronic sialadenitis of the parotid gland. J Oral Rehabil 2009;36(1):2–8.
30. Rice DH. Chronic inflammatory disorders of the salivary glands. Otolaryngol Clin North Am 1999;32(5):813–8.
31. Li NW, Chan WM, Kwan YW, et al. Recurrent parotitis in children. Hong Kong J Paediatr 2011;(16):36–40.
32. Leerdam CM, Martin HC, Issacs D. Recurrent parotitis of childhood. J Paediatr Child Health 2005;41:631–4.
33. Goguen LA, April MM, Karmody CS, et al. Self-induced pneumoparotitis. Arch Otolaryngol Head Neck Surg 1995;121(12):1426–9.
34. Williams MF. Sialolithiasis. Otolaryngol Clin North Am 1999;32(5):819–34.
35. McKenna JP, Bostock DJ, McMenamin PG. Sialolithiasis. Am Fam Physician 1987;36(5):119–25.
36. Peel RL, Seethala RR. Pathology of salivary gland disease. In: Myers EN, Ferris RL, editors. Salivary gland disorders. Berlin: Springer; 2007. p. 33–104.
37. Sunwoo JB, Lewis JS, et al. Malignant neoplasms of the salivary glands. In: Flint PW, editor. Cummings otolaryngology head & neck surgery, vol. 2, 5th edition. Philadelphia: Elsevier Mosby; 2010. p. 1178–99.
38. Eveson JW, Cawson RA. Salivary gland tumours. A review of 2,410 cases with particular reference to histological types, site, age, and sex distribution. J Pathol 1985;146:51–8.
39. Laurie SA. Salivary gland tumors: epidemiology, diagnoses, evaluation, and staging. In: Basow D, editor. UpToDate. Waltham (MA): UpToDate; 2012. Accessed December 17, 2011.
40. Gresham TR, Walner DL, Myer CM. Salivary gland disease in children. In: Flint PW, editor. Cummings otolaryngology head & neck surgery, vol. 2, 5th edition. Philadelphia: Elsevier Mosby; 2010. p. 2850–65.
41. Isaacson GC. Congenital anomalies of the jaw, mouth, oral cavity, and pharynx. In: Basow D, editor. UpToDate. Waltham (MA): UpToDate; 2012. Accessed December 17, 2011.

Emergency Evaluation and Management of the Sore Throat

Angela R. Cirilli, MD, RDMS

KEYWORDS

- Streptococcal pharyngitis • Uvulitis • Infectious mononucleosis • Epiglottitis
- Retropharyngeal abscess • Peritonsillar abscess

KEY POINTS

- The chief complaint of sore throat includes broad differential, including streptococcal pharyngitis, tonsillitis and peritonsillar abscess, retropharyngeal abscess, epiglottitis, uvulitis, and infectious mononucleosis.
- Tonsillitis can be difficult to differentiate from peritonsillar abscess. Ultrasound can help diagnose and direct treatment in these situations.
- In the post vaccine era, epiglottitis is now a disease of adults with insidious onset and more subtle symptoms requiring early aggressive airway management in people presenting with stridor, signs of distress, and systemic disease.
- Uvulitis has infectious and noninfectious causes, which usually respond to medical treatment but occasionally can cause deadly airway obstruction.
- The diagnostic dilemma of streptococcal pharyngitis and mononucleosis continues, and many recommend the aid of laboratory testing in diagnosis and differentiation from other viral causes of pharyngitis before treatment.

INTRODUCTION

The chief complaint of "sore throat" can be caused by conditions ranging from common viral pharyngitis to a deadly diagnosis, such as epiglottitis or severe airway obstruction. A patient with a sore throat should not be taken lightly and deserves your immediate attention, evaluation, and emergent treatment. This article reviews the evaluation, diagnosis, and management of common causes of sore throat: peritonsillar abscess, retropharyngeal abscess, epiglottitis, uvulitis, infectious mononucleosis, and streptococcal pharyngitis.

The author has received no financial support or gifts in preparation of this manuscript.
Department of Emergency Medicine, North Shore University Hospital, Long Island Jewish Hospital, 300 Community Drive, Manhasset, NY 11030, USA
E-mail address: angcirilli@gmail.com

Emerg Med Clin N Am 31 (2013) 501–515
http://dx.doi.org/10.1016/j.emc.2013.01.002
0733-8627/13/$ – see front matter © 2013 Elsevier Inc. All rights reserved.

PERITONSILLAR ABSCESS

Peritonsillar abscess (PTA) is a very common problem, representing 30% of all head and neck abscesses. It is believed to be a complication or progression of another oropharyngeal infection, such as tonsillitis. It is a collection of pus behind the tonsil in the superior arch of the soft palate between the tonsil and the constrictor muscle, previously referred to as "quinsy." It causes significant pain and discomfort. When treated appropriately, with drainage, antibiotics, and pain management, most patients feel significantly better before discharge from the emergency department (ED) and completely recover, with a very low recurrence rate.

Symptoms

The classic presenting symptoms of PTA are as follows:

- Fever
- Malaise
- Dysphagia
- Sore throat
- Drooling
- Muffled or "hot potato" voice
- Referred ear pain

Clinical Examination Findings

Patients typically have inferior medial deviation of the infected tonsil, with uvular deviation away from the affected side. The pharyngeal arch is usually inflamed, erythematous, and enlarged. They may also have lymphadenopathy on the affected side.[1] Trismus, drooling, foul-smelling breath, and a muffled voice are often noted. Peritonsillar abscesses are usually unilateral; however, bilateral occurrences have been described in case reports.[2–4] In bilateral presentations, patients may not have the classic uvular deviation or unilateral prominence, making the clinical diagnosis more difficult and therefore requiring a high degree of suspicion for accurate diagnosis.

Bacterial Causes

The most common bacterial cause is Group A streptococci, usually a complication of preexisting tonsillitis/pharyngitis.[5] Many infections are found to be polymicrobial. Other common causative bacteria are *Streptococcus pyogenes*, *Staphylococcus aureus*, and *Haemophilus influenzae* and anaerobic bacteria, such as *Peptostreptococcus*, *Fusobacterium*, and pigmented *Prevotella*.[1]

Diagnostic Tools

Diagnosis based on the clinical examination findings alone has been shown to have a sensitivity of only 78% and a specificity of 50%. It can be very difficult to differentiate PTA from other causes of sore throat, such as infectious mononucleosis, tonsillar cellulitis, retropharyngeal abscess, and retromolar abscess. In the past, the diagnosis was confirmed with positive aspiration of pus on needle aspiration. More recently, however, imaging, such as ultrasound or computerized tomography (CT), is being used more often. When the physical examination is combined with ultrasound, the sensitivity increases to 89% and the specificity to 100%. CT has been shown to have a sensitivity of 100% and a specificity of 75% in diagnosing PTA.[6] Ultrasound has several advantages over CT: it is easily accessible, has a low cost, and exposes the patient to no radiation, and can be used to guide drainage. The advantage of CT is that it can reveal retropharyngeal or mediastinal fluid collections, indicating extension into the deep neck spaces.

Treatment

PTA is usually treated in an outpatient setting and consists of drainage, antibiotics, steroids, pain control, and intravenous (IV) hydration when necessary. A few patients require hospitalization, when the pain and swelling are so significant that they cannot tolerate fluids or oral antibiotics or if there is a concern about airway stability.

Pharmacologic Treatment

The following medications are typically used:

- Pain control (anti-inflammatory medications, narcotics)
- Antibiotics
- Antipyretics
- Steroids
- IV hydration (when the patient is unable to tolerate liquids)

The use of steroids in addition to IV antibiotics has not been very well studied and remains somewhat controversial. One study, however, demonstrated that use of a single dose of IV steroid plus an antibiotic was statistically superior to antibiotics alone in reducing hours hospitalized, throat pain, fever, and trismus.[7] This study involved hospitalized patients, and a comparison has not been extended to the outpatient setting.

Empiric Antibiotics

Empiric antibiotics should include coverage for Group A streptococci, *S aureus*, and anaerobes. A study performed in the United Kingdom found that administration of penicillin or a cephalosporin plus metronidazole was effective for treatment in 99.2% of patients treated with aspiration and antibiotics in an outpatient ear, nose, and throat (ENT) clinic.[8] Only 1 patient in this series of 118 grew aspirate cultures positive for penicillin-resistant streptococcal species but improved with the use of penicillin plus metronidazole. Empiric regimens for the treatment of PTA are presented in **Box 1**.

Box 1
Empiric regimens for the treatment of peritonsillar abscess

IV treatment

- Ampicillin/sulbactam (Unasyn), 3 g every 6 hours
- Penicillin G, 10 million units every 6 hours, plus metronidazole (Flagyl), 500 mg every 6 hours
- Clindamycin (Cleocin), 900 mg every 8 hours

Oral therapy

- Amoxicillin/clavulanate, 875 mg twice daily
- Penicillin VK, 500 mg 4 times daily, plus metronidazole, 500 mg 4 times daily
- Clindamycin, 600 mg twice daily or 300 mg 4 times daily

Data from Galioto NJ. Peritonsillar abscess, a review. Am Fam Physician 2008;77:199–202.

In areas with an increasing prevalence of methicillin-resistant staphyloccocal infections, clindamycin can be administered intravenously, and vancomycin should be considered if patients fail to improve after 24 hours. For oral administration of antibiotics in areas of high staphylococcal resistance, clindamycin or linezolid can be used.

Surgical Treatment

When a fluid collection is present, antibiotic treatment alone is insufficient for the treatment of PTA. The mainstay of treatment is surgical drainage. Three drainage options are available:

- Emergent "quinsy" tonsillectomy or interval tonsillectomy
- Incision and drainage (performed by an ENT specialist)
- Needle aspiration (blind or guided by ultrasound imaging)

In recent years, incision and drainage and needle aspiration have become favored over tonsillectomy because they can be performed in outpatient settings and EDs, and they avoid the risks associated with general anesthesia and the potential complications of surgery. Emergent tonsillectomy offers no added benefit or effectiveness and is less cost effective than other methods of drainage.[9] Comparisons of incision and drainage with needle aspiration have demonstrated no difference in outcomes with the 2 procedures; however, needle aspiration is easily performed by non-otolaryngologists and is usually less uncomfortable for the patient.[5]

Blind aspiration was used as a diagnostic and therapeutic procedure for PTA. The addition of ultrasound guidance has decreased the number of false-negative drainage procedures In addition, ultrasound is relatively low risk, without complications.[10] It can differentiate tonsillar cellulitis from peritonsillar abscess. Ultrasound guidance also aids in avoiding the dreaded complication of puncture of the carotid artery, which lies in close proximity to the peritonsillar space.

Ultrasound-guided aspiration is typically performed using an endocavitary probe, the size and shape of which are advantageous for insertion into the mouth to look for anechoic fluid collections. Ultrasound will demonstrate a hypoechoic or anechoic fluid collection within or just superior or posterior to the more heterogeneous tonsillar tissue. Color flow can aid in visualization of the carotid artery. Drainage with a 16-gauge or 18-gauge needle can then be performed dynamically, with direct visualization of the needle entering the abscess, or statically after general localization.

RETROPHARYGEAL ABSCESS

Retropharyngeal abscess (RPA) and parapharyngeal abscesses can cause significant morbidity and mortality if they are not detected and treated in a timely manner. Complications include neurologic consequences, extension into the mediastinum and mediastinitis, airway obstruction, sepsis, necrotizing fasciitis, jugular venous thrombosis, and erosion into the carotid artery.

Most cases of RPA occur in children, 80% of them are younger than 5 years old. The reason for the high incidence in this age group might be a retropharyngeal chain of lymph nodes that are susceptible to infection and necrosis and that involute with age.

In adults, RPA tends to occur in people with severe immunocompromise, such as those infected with the human immunodeficiency virus (HIV) or with diabetes or tuberculosis. RPA has also been reported following trauma, such as ingestion of a foreign body (eg, a chicken or fish bone) or following a procedure (eg, insertion of a nasogastric tube, laryngoscopy, or intubation).[11]

Symptoms

The following are common presenting symptoms of RPA:

- Fever
- Neck pain
- Decreased neck movements
- Sore throat/dysphagia
- Palpable neck mass
- Respiratory distress
- Stridor

These symptoms can be vague and nonspecific, especially in the pediatric age group, making the diagnosis difficult. In the patient group analyzed by Grisaru-Soen and colleagues,[12] the most common presenting symptoms were fever and neck pain. Respiratory distress and stridor are rare presenting symptoms, seen in about 5% of patients. These symptoms are more likely to be seen in children younger than 1 year of age, because of the size of the airway. In adults, the presentation is similar, with complaints of dysphagia, sore throat, fever, odynophagia, neck pain, and dyspnea. Adult patients may have bulging, erythema, and edema of the posterior pharyngeal wall (~37%) and nuchal rigidity, stridor, and lymphadenopathy.[11]

Physical Examination

The physical examination may reveal cervical lymphadenopathy, drooling, limitation of neck movement or torticollis, tonsillar hypertrophy, signs of tonsillitis, and a palpable neck mass.

Diagnostic Modalities

RPA is usually diagnosed based on a CT scan. Radiographs can be used as a screening test, and the use of ultrasound is increasing. A typical radiographic finding is widening of more than 5 to 7 mm of the prevertebral soft tissue at the level of the second cervical vertebrae.[13] Air fluid levels in this soft tissue space can also be seen on a radiographic film.

CT findings typically demonstrate a rounded or oval retropharyngeal fluid collection that spreads from side to side and is contained by fascia, with a thick enhancing wall. This fluid collection often displaces the pharynx anteriorly and flattens the prevertebral muscles.[14] Compared with the gold standard of finding a pus collection during surgery, CT has a sensitivity of 81% but a specificity of only 57% for the detection of RPAs.[15]

The use of intraoral ultrasound was described recently for imaging and guided drainage of retropharyngeal abscesses by emergency physicians.[16]

Causes of Infection

Most retropharyngeal abscesses are polymicrobial, including species of *Streptococcus*, *Staphylococcus*, *Neisseria*, and *Haemophilus*. Tuberculosis should be considered in adults who have traveled to regions where it is prevalent and in immunocompromised patients.

Treatment

Nearly all patients with RPA require admission for IV antibiotics, surgical drainage, IV hydration, and pain control.

Antibiotics should be targeted at gram-positive and anaerobic organisms and may include third-generation cephalosporins, expanded-spectrum penicillins, such as ampicillin/sulbactam, and clindamycin, with the addition of vancomycin when staphylococcal resistance is a concern.

There is some controversy regarding the timing for surgical drainage. Some investigators have supported a trial of IV antibiotics alone, with surgery reserved for those failing to respond to medical management after several days. Other investigators, however, support early aggressive management with drainage in the first 24 to 48 hours. Notably, in one study of an aggressive treatment model, neither pus nor abscess was found during surgery in 21% of patients.[17] On analysis, the investigators found that predictive factors for a true abscess requiring drainage included posterior pharyngeal wall bulging, trismus, signs of systemic toxicity, and the size of the collection on CT scan.

Delayed surgical intervention can lead to complications, such as prolonged hospital stay and lymph node rupture into the mediastinum, causing respiratory distress. Therefore, consultation with an otolaryngologist or surgeon is recommended very early in the treatment course.

Outcomes

Coexisting head and neck malignancy, signs of systemic disease, and a C-reactive protein level greater than 100 μg/mL are associated with a higher rate of complications and prolonged hospitalizations in patients with RPA.[18]

EPIGLOTTITIS

Epiglottitis used to be an airway emergency in children, caused by *H influenzae*. Since the introduction of vaccinations, however, its epidemiology and etiology have changed. The overall incidence of epiglottitis has dropped in children and adults, and it is now primarily a disease of adults.

As the epidemiology has shifted, so too have the pathogens. The incidence of epiglottitis caused by other infectious organisms, eg, *S pneumoniae*, has almost tripled since the advent of vaccinations.[19] Infectious causes include *S pyogenes*, *S aureus*, *Moraxella catarrhalis*, *Streptococcus viridans*, *Streptococcus agalactiae*, *Neisseria meningitidis*, *Kingella kingae*, *Bacteroides* species, and the herpes simplex virus.[20]

Symptoms

The classic textbook presentation of a stridorous, febrile, pediatric patient drooling in the tripod position with signs of respiratory distress is no longer very common. Today, epiglottitis most commonly occurs in adults, who have widely varying presentations and symptoms (**Box 2**). It can be very difficult for the emergency care practitioner to identify those who are in danger of impending airway compromise.

In the patient series described by Guardiani and associates,[20] painful swallowing (odynophagia) was the most common symptom, followed by difficulty swallowing and voice changes (in 100%, 85%, and 74%, respectively). Previously accepted classic signs, such as stridor and respiratory distress, were seen in only 13% and 11%, respectively, with the classic tripod positioning seen in only 5%! Surprisingly, 21% of patients in this study required airway intervention.

Treatment

The treatment of epiglottitis includes IV antibiotics, oxygenation, and airway management.

Box 2
Common symptoms of epiglottis

- Pain with swallowing
- Difficulty swallowing
- Voice changes
- Tachycardia
- Drooling
- Fever
- Stridor
- Respiratory distress
- Tripod positioning

Antibiotics for epiglottitis should target the offending gram-positive bacteria: *H influenzae*, *S pyogenes*, and *S pneumoniae*. The chosen medication can include a third-generation cephalosporin, such as ceftriaxone or ampicillin/sulbactam. Levofloxacin or moxifloxacin can be used in patients who are allergic to penicillin.

The value of steroids is unsubstantiated in acute presentations of epiglottitis. Most studies found inconclusive evidence to support their use, as they failed to decrease length of intensive care unit (ICU) stay or duration of intubation. However, Guardiani and associates[20] reported a decreased ICU length of stay in patients who received steroids, but no difference in length of intubation. They recommended that steroids should be considered as an adjunct, but acknowledged that their study involved a small patient population. This question requires further research.

In prevaccination years, when the disease primarily affected children and the need for intubation approached 100%, the recommendation was for early aggressive airway management. In recent years, as the presentation of acute epiglottitis shifted to adults, the intubation rate dropped to 16% to 21%, most likely because adults have larger airways.[20,21]

Now the recommendation is for early aggressive intubation when respiratory distress and stridor are present. Intubation should be performed in the operating room if the patient is stable for transport. For those who are too unstable for transport, awake fiberoptic or nasotracheal intubation is recommended, with a surgeon and an anesthesiologist at the bedside. If intubation is unsuccessful because of a crashing airway and severe airway edema, an emergent tracheostomy or cricothyrotomy should be performed as warranted.

The following are predictive factors for impending but not immediate airway intervention[20]:

- Shortness of breath
- Tachypnea
- Tachycardia
- Rapid onset of symptoms

Patients with these signs and symptoms in the absence of respiratory distress or stridor should be observed in an ICU if intubation is not needed at the time of disposition. Interestingly, drooling and voice changes have not been shown to be predictive of the need for airway intervention.

UVULITIS

Uvulitis (edema of the uvula) is a rare condition with a presentation that can range from benign symptoms to serious airway compromise requiring intubation. Primary isolated angioedema of the uvula is also known as Quinke disease.[22]

Uvulitis has allergic, traumatic, infectious, and neoplastic causes. In addition, it has been reported after the inhalation of marijuana,[23] anesthetic gases, and *Ecbalium elaterium*, a toxic cucumber plant used to treat sinusitis in the Mediterranean region.[24] Traumatic causes include intubation, endoscopy, and aggressive oral suctioning.[25] Infectious sources are less common and include bacteria, such as group A streptococci, *H influenzae*, and *S pneumoniae*.

The cause of uvulitis can usually be elucidated through the clinical history. Infectious causes should be suspected when the patient has an elevated white blood cell count and fever. When infection is suspected, the physician should also have a high suspicion for concomitant epiglottitis, tonsillitis, and pharyngitis. Under these circumstances, many investigators support imaging or radiography of the neck as part of the assessment for impending airway compromise and edema.[26]

Presenting symptoms usually include sore throat, foreign body sensation, dysphagia, drooling, stridor, a gagging sensation that is worse with lying supine, and muffled or "hot potato" voice. Pain, fever, and odynophagia suggest an infectious source. Examination will reveal an enlarged and erythematous uvula, often with contiguous tonsillitis, pharyngitis, or cellulitis. In patients with angioedema, the uvula is enlarged, boggy, and nonerythematous, appearing like a large pale grape. If the patient has hereditary angioedema, the soft palate may be enlarged and edematous as well.[27]

The treatment of uvular edema matches classic treatments for allergic reactions, including dexamethasone, antihistamines such as diphenhydramine, as well as intramuscular injection of epinephrine. The administration of nebulized β-agonists and racemic epinephrine has also been described. Pain control with IV narcotics is often necessary. Topical application of lidocaine and epinephrine has been described in case reports. IV antibiotics are reserved for patients in whom an infectious source is suspected, those with severe presentations, and, in many cases, for children, in whom uvulitis is often associated with infection.

Airway protection is the most serious consideration when managing a patient with uvulitis. Preparation for intubation should include having equipment at the bedside; however, many patients with dramatic or severe initial presentations do well with IV medication and management in addition to observation and do not require intubation. When airway compromise seems imminent, consultation with an ENT specialist is recommended for evaluation of supra-epiglottic or laryngeal involvement.

INFECTIOUS MONONUCLEOSIS

Infectious mononucleosis is a flulike syndrome with associated pharyngitis. It is caused by the Epstein-Barr virus (EBV), which is believed to be passed via oral secretion (hence the name "kissing disease"). Its prevalence is somewhat unknown and varies by geographic location throughout the world. The presentation of acute EBV infection varies widely based on age and the immune competence of the host. Because of these variables, diagnosis can be difficult.

An acute infection tends to be missed in younger children, as it is often less dramatic than the presentation in adults. Signs and symptoms progress in severity with the age of the host.[28] The range of severity can be very mild (eg, a coldlike illness in a young child) to severe disease in an adult, with the potential for complications and even death from splenomegaly and rupture, airway obstruction, meningoencephalitis, hemolytic anemia, or thrombocytopenia, all of which occur in as few as 1% of those infected.[29] In less developed countries, the infection is more common in younger children, which could be explained by crowding and transmission of the virus through saliva on toys, hands, bottles, and utensils. In the United States, the classic infection is more common in younger adults and adolescents.

Patient History

Infectious mononucleosis has an incubation period of 4 to 6 weeks, and it can be shed by a recovering host intermittently for months after an acute infection. Therefore, contact with someone with a similar illness is often difficult to track. Patients often describe a syndrome of the worst sore throat they have ever experienced, along with fatigue, fever, headache, abdominal discomfort, and lack of appetite (**Box 3**). The 3 most common symptoms of infectious mononucleosis (ie, sore throat, fatigue, and headache) match those of cervical lymphadenopathy.[30] The patient's temperature usually is at its highest for 5 to 7 days, then it gradually declines toward normal. The symptoms of acute mononucleosis can last longer than those of many other viral infections (up to 16 days), and fatigue may linger weeks or months.

Clinical Findings/Physical Examination

The physical examination findings of cervical lymphadenopathy (affecting both posterior and anterior nodes), pharyngitis, and fever are found in most patients (75%–100%).[31] Less common findings include palpable hepatomegaly or splenomegaly, eyelid edema, arthralgia, myalgia, somnolence, and a maculopapular rash (often associated with the recent start of an antibiotic for bacterial pharyngitis). The signs and symptoms are as follows, in order of reported prevalence:

- Cervical lymphadenopathy
- Fatigue
- Pharyngitis/exudative tonsillitis
- Fever
- Splenomegaly
- Hepatomegaly

Tonsillitis due to mononucleosis can be difficult to distinguish from other forms of tonsillopharyngitis, such as those caused by streptococci, or viral causes, such as herpetic infections and cytomegalovirus. Therefore, findings from the physical examination alone are not reliable enough to make the diagnosis.

Box 3	
Prevalence of symptoms of infectious mononucleosis	
Sore throat	95%
Fatigue	90%
Headache	75%
Fever	70%
Body aches	50%
Decreased appetite	50%
Abdominal discomfort	40%

Data from Son KH, Shin MY. Clinical features of Epstein-Barr virus-associated infectious mononucleosis in hospitalized Korean children. Korean J Pediatr 2011;54(10):409–13.

Diagnosis

Mononucleosis is difficult to diagnose because its presentation is similar to that of many other viral and bacterial causes of a sore throat. The prolonged length of symptoms and severe fatigue can be considered indicators.

Laboratory Findings

Abnormalities on certain laboratory tests, such as mildly elevated transaminases and leukocytosis, can point toward the diagnosis. Leukocytosis is defined as a predominance of lymphocytes greater than 50%, with the presence of atypical lymphocytes.

Diagnostic laboratory tests specific for mononucleosis include immunoassay testing for immunoglobulin (Ig)G and IgM antibodies for the viral capsid antigen of EBV and the absence of EBV nuclear antigen. Very early in the infection, detection of EBV by real-time polymerase chain reaction and measurement of direct EBV viral load can be useful and as sensitive as 100%.[32] The heterophile antibody, or monospot, test is a latex agglutination assay of horse red blood cells, which detects antibodies to EBV. It can be falsely negative if the test is performed too early in the infection, because the antibody level peaks about 2 weeks after the primary infection. False-positive monospot tests have been reported, although rarely, in association with conditions such as toxoplasmosis, herpes simplex infections, HIV infection, and lymphoma.

Treatment

The treatment for infectious mononucleosis is largely supportive. Fever control and pain management with nonsteroidal anti-inflammatory drugs and acetaminophen constitute the mainstay of treatment. The use of steroids to help with symptom management has been studied, but this approach has not proven to shorten the course of the illness or prevent serious complications. The adverse effects of steroids in patients with mononucleosis have not been adequately studied.[33] Antivirals have been shown to inhibit EBV replication in vitro, but one recent meta-analysis of use of acyclovir failed to show any benefit.[33]

Complications

The median duration of symptoms is 16 days.[29] Most persons infected with EBV have resolution of symptoms within 1 month after their onset, with resolution of transaminitis.[31] Chronic fatigue has been described as a complication of infectious mononucleosis, but that relationship is unclear.

Splenic rupture is the most feared and most common fatal complication of mononucleosis. Fortunately, it is relatively rare, being reported in only 0.1% to 0.5% of patients with infectious mononucleosis. Most patients require splenectomy in the setting of hemodynamic instability. Conservative treatment has been advocated for hemodynamically stable patients, but this approach is somewhat controversial.[34] Splenic rupture is believed to happen from rupture of the capsule secondary to an underlying expanding hematoma or from the pressure of the diaphragm against the spleen during Valsalva maneuver, such as coughing or vomiting.

Other very rare complications include airway obstruction secondary to severe tonsillar hypertrophy, meningitis, encephalitis, myocarditis, hemolytic anemia, and thrombocytopenia.

To help prevent complications (particularly splenic rupture), individuals recovering from mononucleosis are encouraged to refrain from strenuous activities. This includes avoiding participation in sports until all symptoms of the acute infection resolve (usually about a month). Ultrasound imaging can be considered as a means of evaluating for splenomegaly in patients who are eager to resume their pre-illness physical activities.[35]

STREPTOCOCCAL PHARYNGITIS

Group A streptococcal pharyngitis (GAS pharyngitis) is the most common manifestation of bacterial pharyngitis/tonsillitis. It is presents in up to 37% of all children presenting with a sore throat to an outpatient clinic or ED and 24% of those presenting at younger than 5 years.[36] It is most common in children between the ages of 5 and 15 years and occurs more commonly in the winter and spring. The diagnosis of streptococcal pharyngitis has been studied extensively, as it can have serious long-term outcomes, such as rheumatic fever, heart disease, and poststreptococcal glomerulonephritis. It is also very difficult to distinguish from nonbacterial causes of tonsillitis and pharyngitis.

Clinical Manifestations

The following are the common symptoms of GAS pharyngitis[37]:

- Sore throat
- Dysphagia
- Fever
- Headache
- Abdominal pain
- Nausea
- Vomiting

The fever usually resolves within 3 to 5 days, and sore throat is self-limited, resolving within 1 week.[38]

Physical Examination

The following are common physical examination findings:

- Pharyngeal erythema
- Palatal petechiae
- Uvular inflammation/uvulitis
- Anterior cervical lymphadenopathy
- Tonsillar exudates
- Rash (scarlet fever)

Scarlet fever is an erythematous, blanching, papular rash that feels like "fine sandpaper" on palpation. The rash may desquamate as it dissipates. To differentiate scarlet fever from viral pharyngitis, patients should have the absence of viral symptoms, such as a cough, runny nose, and a hoarse voice, and lack of conjunctivitis.

Diagnostic Criteria

The Centor criteria constitute the best known scoring system to aid in the diagnosis of pharyngitis in adults, and it has been modified for application to children. The Centor scoring system assigns 1 point for each of following:

- Fever >38°C
- Absence of cough
- Tender anterior cervical nodes
- Tonsillar exudates

These criteria are used to predict the likelihood of a positive culture for GAS pharyngitis in adults. Scores range from 0 to 4, with probabilities from 2.5% to 56.0%.[39] In a recent study, the presence of all 4 Centor criteria gave an overall positive predictive value of 47.9%; the value fell to 41.6% when 3 criteria were present.[40]

Laboratory Testing

The rapid streptococcal antigen tests are widely available and have been used and studied extensively as an adjunct to making the diagnosis of GAS pharyngitis. Specificity for the test has been reported to be as high as 95%, with a sensitivity of 80% to 90%.[38] Throat cultures are much more sensitive, between 90% and 95%; however, they require up to 48 hours for results.

Treatment

The treatment of GAS pharyngitis consists of antibiotics to avoid suppurative and rheumatic complications in addition to pain and fever control. The Infectious Diseases Society of America (IDSA) recommends a 10-day course of any of the following oral antibiotics[40]:

- Penicillin V, 250 mg twice a day or 3 times a day for children, and 3 or 4 times a day for adults
- Erythromycin
- First-generation cephalosporin

An alternative to oral antibiotics is intramuscular benzathine penicillin G. It is given as a single dose and can be used for patients who do not tolerate oral liquids well. Amoxicillin suspension is often used in place of penicillin for children because it tastes better.

Testing Guidelines

Several strategies have been proposed to guide antibiotic prescribing and laboratory testing for GAS, but they are poorly adhered to by practitioners and may vary widely when applied to various geographic regions of the world. Much confusion exists because recommendations vary greatly among the American College of Physicians (ACP), the American Academy of Family Physicians (AAFP), the Centers for Disease Control and Prevention (CDC), the IDSA, and the American Heart Association.[41] The consensus among them is clear that, when scoring reveals none of the symptoms suggestive of GAS pharyngitis or when the Centor criteria score is 0, no testing or treatment is necessary. They vary, however, when patients have a few or all of the symptoms in the scoring system. The ACP, AAFP, and CDC recommend different strategies for treating patients with all 4 Centor criteria, those who have 3 Centor criteria and a positive rapid test, and those who have 3 criteria but in whom no test was done. The IDSA disagrees with this strategy because, in the organization's view, it will result in overprescribing.

McIsaac and associates[42] analyzed the treatment strategies that combine Centor criteria, rapid tests, and cultures. They concluded that, based on scoring systems alone, treating those with a modified Centor score of 3 or more without rapid assay or culture testing would result in 60% of patients continuing unnecessary antibiotics and 40% receiving an unnecessary prescription. In summary, many agree that in patients with only 1 or 2 Centor criteria, a rapid test should be performed, a culture should be added if results are negative, and patients with positive results should be treated. Additional testing when the score is 3 or 4 is controversial. There is consensus that, when used appropriately, a positive rapid test or culture does identify patients who should be treated.

SUMMARY

The differential diagnosis of a patient presenting with a sore throat is very broad and encompasses peritonsillar abscess, RPA, epiglottitis, uvulitis, infectious mononucleosis, and streptococcal pharyngitis. These diagnoses can be very difficult to differentiate from one another. A high level of clinical suspicion and a detailed physical examination with additional testing as necessary are required to appropriately diagnose and treat these conditions. Although a sore throat can be as mild as the common cold or viral pharyngitis, it could be an indicator of a life-threatening problem, an ensuing airway obstruction, or an omen of a very difficult airway should intubation be necessary. Therefore, all cases should be taken seriously until appropriate evaluation, history, and testing are completed.

REFERENCES

1. Galioto NJ. Peritonsillar abscess, a review. Am Fam Physician 2008;77(2): 199–202.
2. Pham V, Gungor A. Bilateral peritonsillar abscess: case report and literature review. Am J Otolaryngol 2012;33:163–7.
3. Papacharalampous GX, Vlastarakos PV, Kotsis G, et al. Bilateral peritonsillar abscesses: a case presentation and review of the current literature with regard to the controversies in diagnosis and treatment. Case Report Med 2011;2011: 981924.
4. Fasano CJ, Chudnofsky C, Vanderbeek P. Bilateral peritonsillar abscesses: not your usual sore throat. J Emerg Med 2005;29(1):45–7.
5. Johnson RF, Stewart MG, Wright CC. An evidence-based review of the treatment of peritonsillar abscess. Otolaryngol Head Neck Surg 2003;128(3):332–43.
6. Scott PM, Loftus WK, Kew J, et al. Diagnosis of peritonsillar infections: a prospective study of ultrasound, computerized tomography and clinical diagnosis. J Laryngol Otol 1999;113(3):229–32.
7. Ozbek C, Aygenc E, Tuna EU, et al. Use of steroids in the treatment of peritonsillar abscess. J Laryngol Otol 2004;118(6):439–42.
8. Repanos C, Mukherjee P, Alwahab YJ. Role of microbiological studies in management of peritonsillar abscess. J Laryngol Otol 2009;123(8):877–9.
9. Khayr W, Taepke J. Management of peritonsillar abscess: needle aspiration versus incision and drainage versus tonsillectomy. Am J Ther 2005;12(4):344–50.
10. Lyon M, Blaivas M. Intraoral ultrasound in the diagnosis and treatment of suspected peritonsillar abscess in the emergency department. Acad Emerg Med 2005;12(1):85–8.
11. Harkani A, Hassani R, Ziad T, et al. Retropharyngeal abscess in adults: five case reports and review of the literature. ScientificWorldJournal 2011;11:1623–9.
12. Grisaru-Soen G, Komisar O, Aizenstein O, et al. Retropharyngeal and parapharyngeal abscess in children—epidemiology, clinical features and treatment. Int J Pediatr Otorhinolaryngol 2010;74(9):1016–20.
13. McLeod C, Stanley K. Images in emergency medicine: retropharyngeal abscess. West J Emerg Med 2008;9:55.
14. Hoang JK, Branstetter B IV, Eastwood JD, et al. Multiplanar CT and MRI of collections in the retropharyngeal space: is it an abscess? AJR Am J Roentgenol 2011; 196(4):W426–32.

15. Daya H, Lo S, Papsin BC, et al. Retropharyngeal and parapharyngeal infections in children: the Toronto experience. Int J Pediatr Otorhinolaryngol 2005;69(1):81–6.

16. Blaivas M, Adhikari S. Bedside transoral ultrasonographically guided drainage of a retropharyngeal abscess in the emergency department. Ann Emerg Med 2011; 58(5):497–8.

17. Page N, Bauer EM, Lieu J. Clinical features and treatment of retropharyngeal abscess in children. Otolaryngol Head Neck Surg 2008;138:300–6.

18. Wang LF, Tai CF, Kuo WR, et al. Predisposing factors of complicated deep neck infections: 12-year experience at a single institution. J Otolaryngol Head Neck Surg 2010;39(4):335–41.

19. Isakson M, Hugosson S. Acute epiglottitis: epidemiology and Streptococcus pneumoniae serotype distribution in adults. J Laryngol Otol 2011;125:390–3.

20. Guardiani E, Bliss M, Harley E. Supraglottitis in the era following widespread immunization against Haemophilus influenzae Type B: evolving principles in diagnosis and management. Laryngoscope 2010;120:2183–8.

21. Price IM, Preyra I, Fernandes C, et al. Adult epiglottitis: a five-year retrospective chart review in a major urban centre. EM Advances. CJEM 2005;7(6):387–90.

22. Johnson W, Shastri N, Fowler M. Quincke's disease. West J Emerg Med 2011; 12(4):370.

23. Boyce S, Quigley M. Uvulitis and partial upper airway obstruction following cannabis inhalation. Emerg Med (Fremantle) 2002;14:106–8.

24. Kokkonouzis I, Antoniou G. Images in emergency medicine: uvular oedema caused by intranasal aspiration of undiluted juice of Ecbalium elaterium. Emerg Med J 2009;26(8):566.

25. Gilmore T, Mirin M. Traumatic uvulitis from a suction catheter. J Emerg Med 2012; 43:e479–80.

26. Jerrard DA, Olshaker J. Simultaneous uvulitis and epiglottitis without fever or leukocytosis. Am J Emerg Med 1996;14(6):551–2.

27. Goldberg R, Lawton R, Newton E, et al. Evaluation and management of acute uvular edema. Ann Emerg Med 1993;22(2):251–5.

28. Son KH, Shin MY. Clinical features of Epstein-Barr virus-associated infectious mononucleosis in hospitalized Korean children. Korean J Pediatr 2011;54(10): 409–13.

29. Odumade OA, Hogquist KA, Balfour HH Jr. Progress and problems in under-standing and managing primary Epstein-Barr virus infections. Clin Microbiol Rev 2011;24:193–209.

30. Macsween KF, Higgins CD, McAulay KA, et al. Infectious mononucleosis in university students in the United Kingdom: evaluation of the clinical features and consequences of the disease. Clin Infect Dis 2010;50(5):699–706.

31. Rea TD, Russo JE, Katon W, et al. Prospective study of the natural history of infectious mononucleosis caused by Epstein-Barr virus. J Am Board Fam Pract 2001; 14(4):234–42.

32. Vouloumanou EK, Rafailidis PI, Falagas ME. Current diagnosis and management of infectious mononucleosis. Curr Opin Hematol 2012;19(1):14–20.

33. Torre D, Tambini R. Acyclovir for treatment of infectious mononucleosis: a meta-analysis. Scand J Infect Dis 1999;31:543–7.

34. Asgari MM, Begos DG. Spontaneous splenic rupture in infectious mononucleosis: a review. Yale J Biol Med 1997;70(2):175–82.

35. O'Connor TE, Skinner LJ, Kiely P, et al. Return to contact sports following infectious mononucleosis: the role of serial ultrasonography. Ear Nose Throat J 2011;90(8):21–4.

36. Shaikh N, Leonard E, Martin JM. Prevalence of streptococcal pharyngitis and streptococcal carriage in children: a meta-analysis. Pediatrics 2010;126(3):e557.
37. Langlois D, Andreae M. Group A streptococcal infections. Pediatr Rev 2011; 32(10):423–30.
38. Bisno A, Gerber M, Gwaltney J, et al. Practice guidelines for the diagnosis and management of Group A streptococcal pharyngitis. Clin Infect Dis 2002;35: 113–25.
39. Centor RM, Witherspoon JM, Dalton HP, et al. The diagnosis of strep throat in adults in the emergency room. Med Decis Making 1981;1:239–46.
40. Wagner F, Mathiason M. Using Centor criteria to diagnose streptococcal pharyngitis. Nurse Pract 2008;33(9):10–2.
41. Wessels MR. Clinical practice: streptococcal pharyngitis. N Engl J Med 2011; 364(7):648–55.
42. McIsaac WJ, Kellner JD, Aufricht P, et al. Empirical validation of guidelines for the management of pharyngitis in children and adults. JAMA 2004;291(13):1587–95.

Regional Nerve Blocks of the Face

Joshua B. Moskovitz, MD, MPH*, Frank Sabatino, MD

KEYWORDS

- Peripheral nerve block • Regional nerve block • Facial anesthesia • Analgesia

KEY POINTS

- V1 nerve blocks anesthetize the forehead and much of the anterior scalp and are underutilized in repairs.
- V2 nerve blocks are quick and easy and are especially useful in this cosmetically high-risk area. Maxillary nerve blocks allow anesthesia without making wounds edematous and ease repairs.
- V3 nerve blocks are especially convenient in lower lip lacerations.
- Auricular blocks are vital in this dense low-volume area that makes local anesthesia especially difficult.
- Nasal blocks are useful in lacerations and relocations of fractures.

For repair of lacerations on the face, regional nerve blocks offer a multitude of benefits: longer-lasting analgesia, less discomfort because fewer injections are needed and they can be placed in less sensitive areas, and improved cosmesis because the wound margins are less distorted compared with the use of local infiltration. Patients understandably object to the multiple injections that are required to achieve sufficient analgesia through local infiltration. Additionally, anyone who has sutured a wound on a patient's face will recall the difficulties of aligning the margins of an edematous wound after injecting a local anesthetic. This article presents a review of the network that innervates the face and describes the induction of nerve blocks for specific areas.

The medications typically used to induce facial anesthesia are lidocaine, 1%, with or without epinephrine; bupivacaine, 0.25% to 0.5%, with or without epinephrine; and topical lidocaine, epinephrine, tetracaine (LET). In general, local infiltration of lidocaine provides 1 to 2 hours of analgesia, which can be extended to 2 to 4 hours with the addition of epinephrine. The maximum dose for plain lidocaine is 4.5 mg/kg (up to 300 mg total). For lidocaine with epinephrine, the dose increases up to 7 mg/kg (500 mg total). In practical terms, for a 70 kg patient, that translates into 30 mL of

---

Department of Emergency Medicine, North Shore University Hospital, Hofstra North Shore-Long Island Jewish School of Medicine, 300 Community Drive, Manhasset, NY 11030, USA
* Corresponding author.
E-mail address: joshmoskovitz@gmail.com

Emerg Med Clin N Am 31 (2013) 517–527
http://dx.doi.org/10.1016/j.emc.2013.01.003
0733-8627/13/$ – see front matter emed.theclinics.com

1% plain lidocaine, or 50 mL of 1% lidocaine with epinephrine. Bupivacaine provides 4 to 8 hours of analgesia; the addition of epinephrine increases the duration to 8 to 16 hours of relief.[1] When bupivacaine is used, a concentration of 0.25% is typical, with a 2.5 mg/kg safety limit in adults and a 2 mg/kg safety limit in children.[2] For large or multiple wounds, the total amount of anesthetic required if using local infiltration can exceed safe limits and lead to toxicity, making the use of nerve blocks essential.

LET is used predominantly in children, but it also has utility when suturing a wound in an adult, especially in areas that are difficult to anesthetize because they cross midlines and cutaneous nerve regions. In preparation for the repair of a small laceration across the nose, a quick smudge of LET can achieve a proper anesthetic level to allow wound closure without the discomfort of an injection.

Performing nerve blocks of the face is a skill that can be learned easily and quickly. Paoli and colleagues[3] trained dermatologists with no previous experience to induce nerve blocks through a 4-hour course consisting of video demonstration and hands-on training; all of the participants reported skill retention at 1- and 2-year follow-up.

ANATOMY OF FACIAL NERVES

The nerves that provide sensation to the face originate as cranial nerve (CN) V. Its main sensory nucleus is in the midpons, with extension caudally as the spinal nucleus and rostrally as the mesencephalic nucleus.[4]

CN V then divides into 3 main roots. Division 1 covers sensation from the upper eyes throughout the forehead and parts of the nose; division 2 covers sensation from underneath the eyes to the upper lip and laterally, and division 3 covers sensation from the chin to the lower lip, then up and around the face.[5] Each division of CN V has further subdivisions, where peripheral blocks are targeted to achieve proper analgesia.

The ophthalmic nerve (CN V_1) splits off the trigeminal ganglia, where its main branch, the frontal nerve, dives through the orbital cavity, producing 2 main sensory nerves of the face, the supraorbital and supratrochlear nerves.[6] The supraorbital nerve exits the frontal bone through the supraorbital foramen and provides sensation to the superior aspects of the eye and the forehead and, extending posteriorly, provides cutaneous coverage to a large portion of the scalp.[6] The supratrochlear nerve exits the skull medially to the supraorbital nerve and sensates more medial aspects of the forehead and anterior portions of the scalp. Lastly, the nasociliary nerve branches off the ophthalmic nerve, giving rise to the small infratrochlear nerve that provides sensation to the superior medial aspect of the eyelid inferior to the brow. The last sensation provided by CN V_1 is via the external nasal branch of the anterior ethmoidal nerve, sensating the medial portion of the nares.

The maxillary nerve (CN V_2) branches off the trigeminal nerve, diving through the foramen rotundum.[6] The zygomatic nerve branches off the main bundle, terminating in the zygomaticotemporal and zygomaticofacial nerves. The zygomaticofacial nerve exits the skull at its foramen laterally and inferior to the orbit, providing cutaneous sensation to its small local area. The zygomaticotemporal nerve extends along the temples, providing superior lateral sensation via CN V_2. The major sensation of CN V_2 is via the infraorbital nerve exiting its foramen and splitting in all directions. The infraorbital nerve sensates the lower eyelids, the lateral nares, and the superior lip areas.

The mandibular nerve (CN V_3) branches off the trigeminal nerve, traveling inferiorly through foramen ovale, where it splits into the anterior and posterior divisions.[6] The primary relevance is with the posterior division, which gives rise to the inferior alveolar, lingual, and auriculotemporal nerves. The lingual nerve terminates as the sublingual nerve, and the inferior alveolar terminates as the mental nerve. The auriculotemporal nerve splits off the posterior branch, exiting anterior to the ear and posterior to the neck of the mandible between portions of the parotid gland, traveling superiorly up to the temples, supplying sensation to those areas of the face. The remaining portion of the posterior division divides into the inferior alveolar and the lingual nerves. The inferior alveolar nerve enters the mandibular foramen and provides sensation to all of its respective inferior dentition. Anteriorly, it exits the mandible through the lateral of midline mental foramen, providing sensation to the anterior mandible as the mental nerve. The lingual nerve terminates as the sublingual nerve within the oral cavity in the anterior portions of the mandible. Of notable mention is the buccal nerve, which branches off the anterior division, providing sensation to the buccal mucosa between the superior and inferior teeth.

The great auricular, transverse cervical, greater occipital, lesser occipital, and great auricular cervical plexus nerves are not part of the trigeminal nerve (CN V), but they need to be considered in the sensation of the head. These nerves predominantly arise off the cervical plexus as collaborations of multiple cervical nerves.[6] The great auricular nerve courses inferiorly to the ear, with some anterior sensation and inferior dorsal sensation. The lesser occipital nerve courses posterior to the auricle, and the greater occipital nerve provides even further posterior sensation to the scalp.

APPLICATION OF NERVE BLOCKS

Nerve blocks should always be performed in a safe and judicious manner. Proper technique for a percutaneous approach includes the preparation of the skin by disinfecting prior to skin puncture. If an intraoral or mucosal membrane approach is being used, a topical anesthetic should be applied prior to puncture. Safe doses of medication must be calculated. Before any infiltration of drug, correct needle placement should be verified with aspiration, because blood vessels run in close proximity to the target nerves.

Laceration of the Forehead/Eyebrows/Eyelids

The supraorbital nerve is blocked at the notch where it exits the skull. This large nerve (along with the supratrochlear and infratrochlear nerves) provides sensation over a large distribution of the forehead, extending posteriorly to the distal scalp (**Fig. 1**). The supraorbital notch can be located by placing the thumb of the nondominant hand on the superior orbital rim. With the syringe in the dominant hand, one should inject a small wheal of anesthetic agent just lateral to the notch, and then advance approximately 2 cm until past the medial canthus. One should then inject 1 to 2 mL there, and an additional 2 to 3 mL while withdrawing the needle (**Fig. 2**).[7]

The lacrimal nerve provides sensation to the lateral and medial thirds of the eyelid (**Fig. 3**). This nerve must be blocked (along with the supraorbital) in order to repair most eyelid lacerations. One should inject at the edge of the superior orbital rim, directly up from the lateral canthus (**Fig. 4**).[8] Alternatively, an injection along the entire superior orbital rim can be used to anesthetize all the aforementioned nerves.

Laceration of the Nose

One should anesthetize the nose with multiple individual blocks, giving careful consideration of crossing midline sensation. Nasal blocks can be induced by targeting the aforementioned infratrochlear nerve for inferior lateral aspects of the nose and the

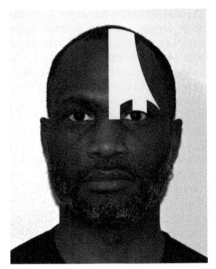

Fig. 1. Supraorbital, supratrochlear, and infratrochlear nerve distribution. (*Courtesy of* Alisa Gibson, MD, DMD. University of Maryland School of Medicine, Baltimore, MD.)

supratrochlear nerve for superior aspects. The dorsal nasal nerve requires a separate block to provide analgesia for the tip and mid-distal portions of the nose (**Fig. 5**). This nerve exits approximately 6 to 10 mm from the midline of the nasal bones, and is best targeted there. One should palpate the transition between the nasal bones and cartilage using the thumb on 1 side and the index finger on the other. One should inject 1 to 2 mL at that point (**Fig. 6**).[8]

Laceration of the Infraorbital Area

For repair of a laceration to the midface or upper lip (**Fig. 7**), the infraorbital nerve can easily be blocked. There are 2 possible approaches, either extraoral or intraoral. The extraoral approach requires palpating the infraorbital ridge to locate the infraorbital foramen, where the nerve exits the skull. The foramen is located on a line dropped

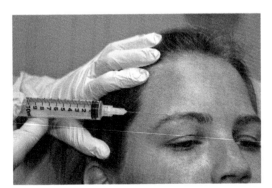

Fig. 2. Supraorbital, supratrochlear, and infratrochlear nerve block. (*Courtesy of* Alisa Gibson, MD, DMD. University of Maryland School of Medicine, Baltimore, MD.)

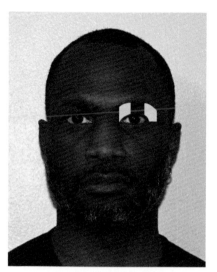

Fig. 3. Lacrimal nerve distribution. (*Courtesy of* Alisa Gibson, MD, DMD. University of Maryland School of Medicine, Baltimore, MD.)

from the medial limbus; it opens approximately 5 mm below the orbital rim along that line. One should infiltrate local anesthetic at this location (taking care to not enter the foramen itself) (**Fig. 8**). The intraoral approach entails pulling the upper lip out with the thumb and placing 1 finger on the infraorbital ridge externally. With the other hand, one should advance the needle intraorally in a superior direction toward the foramen. Once bone is contacted, one should withdraw slightly and inject 3 to 4 mL (**Fig. 9**).[7]

Laceration of the Mandible/Lower Lip

Mental nerve block provides anesthesia to the lower lip, to the level of the labiomental fold (**Fig. 10**), but lacerations near the midline may require bilateral blocks due to the cross-innervation of the sensory fibers. One should palpate the mental foramen, which is located near the apices of the premolars. One should then direct the needle

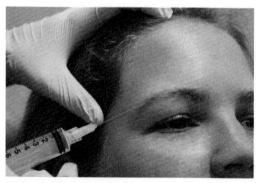

Fig. 4. Lacrimal nerve block. (*Courtesy of* Alisa Gibson, MD, DMD. University of Maryland School of Medicine, Baltimore, MD.)

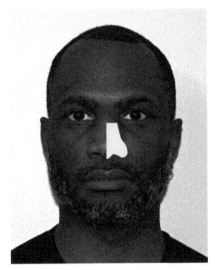

Fig. 5. Dorsal nasal nerve distribution. (*Courtesy of* Alisa Gibson, MD, DMD. University of Maryland School of Medicine, Baltimore, MD.)

downward while retracting the lower lip and inject 3 to 4 mL directly over the foramen (**Fig. 11**).[8]

Sensation to the chin pad inferior to the labiomental fold is provided by the nerve to the mylohyoid. Addition of the mental plus block is frequently necessary to repair wounds to the chin. Just like the mental nerve block, bilateral blocks are generally required. To perform this block, the needle is inserted in the same location near the mental foramen, but directed anteriorly instead of toward the bone. One should advance the needle to just past the inferior mandibular border (almost out of the skin), and inject 1 to 2 mL.[8]

Inferior Alveolar Nerve Block

Achieving regional block of the inferior alveolar nerve is 1 of the most rewarding in regard to providing immediate and continued pain relief, but it is also the most

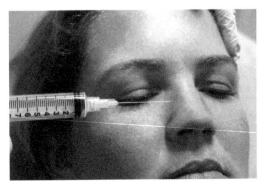

Fig. 6. Dorsal nasal nerve block. (*Courtesy of* Alisa Gibson, MD, DMD. University of Maryland School of Medicine, Baltimore, MD.)

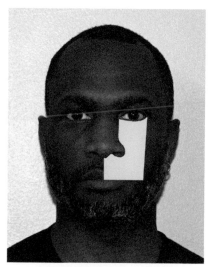

Fig. 7. Infraorbital nerve distribution. (*Courtesy of* Alisa Gibson, MD, DMD. University of Maryland School of Medicine, Baltimore, MD.)

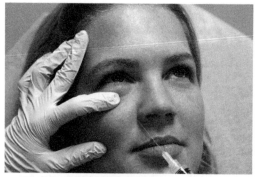

Fig. 8. Infraorbital nerve block—extraoral approach. (*Courtesy of* Alisa Gibson, MD, DMD. University of Maryland School of Medicine, Baltimore, MD.)

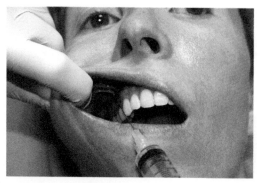

Fig. 9. Infraorbital nerve block—intraoral approach. (*Courtesy of* Alisa Gibson, MD, DMD. University of Maryland School of Medicine, Baltimore, MD.)

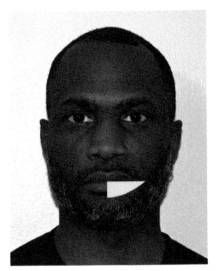

Fig. 10. Mental nerve distribution. (*Courtesy of* Alisa Gibson, MD, DMD. University of Maryland School of Medicine, Baltimore, MD.)

challenging. Failure rates on the first attempt of up to 15% to 20% have been seen, even in experienced hands,[9] so repeating the block is completely reasonable and frequently necessary. Understanding the anatomy is key to effective performance of this block. The nerve is best accessed where it exits through the inferior alveolar canal. The canal is located approximately 1 cm above the mandibular occlusal plane, anterior to the pterygomandibular raphe (**Fig. 12**). One should use the thumb of the nondominant hand to retract the cheek. The tissue must be pulled taut. The syringe should be held parallel to the mandibular occlusal plane, with the barrel overlying the premolars opposite the side being anesthetized. It may be helpful to bend the needle slightly. One should aim toward the inferior alveolar canal. A standard 27-guage needle will need to be inserted approximately 75% of its length, or 20 to 25 mm. Bone (mandibular ramus) must be contacted at that depth, or failure is a near certainty. Aspiration is imperative.

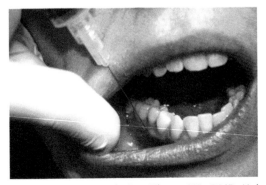

Fig. 11. Mental nerve block. (*Courtesy of* Alisa Gibson, MD, DMD. University of Maryland School of Medicine, Baltimore, MD.)

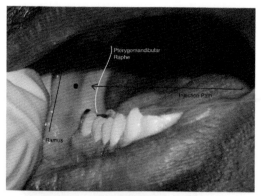

Fig. 12. Intraoral nerve anatomy and approach. (*Courtesy of* Alisa Gibson, MD, DMD. University of Maryland School of Medicine, Baltimore, MD.)

The inferior alveolar artery runs directly with the nerve, so blood return is actually a positive indication that nerve has been located. One should simply withdraw slightly (no more than 1 mm) and aspirate again, then inject 4 to 5 mL.[10]

Laceration of the Ear

The ear is anesthetized through ring-like blocks around it. One should insert the needle 1 cm inferior to the attachment of the earlobe to the scalp, then direct the needle toward the tragus, aspirate, and inject while pulling back. The needle should not be completely removed. It should be redirected posteriorly, along the direction of the helix. One should aspirate and inject as one pulls back again. This will provide inferior sensation relief. A similar procedure is used for the superior portion. The needle should be inserted approximately 1 cm superior to the attachment of the ear to the scalp. One

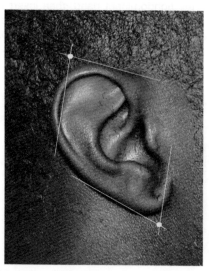

Fig. 13. Ear ring block. (*Courtesy of* Alisa Gibson, MD, DMD. University of Maryland School of Medicine, Baltimore, MD.)

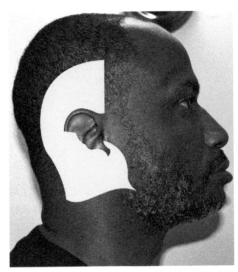

Fig. 14. Greater auricular and lesser occipital nerve distribution. (*Courtesy of* Alisa Gibson, MD, DMD. University of Maryland School of Medicine, Baltimore, MD.)

should direct the needle toward the tragus, aspirate, and inject while pulling back. One should redirect posteriorly, along the direction of the helix, then aspirate, and once again inject while pulling back (**Fig. 13**).[11]

Posterior Head/Scalp

The greater auricular and lesser occipital nerves provide sensation to the skin posterior and inferior to the ear, as well as to the pinna and lower two-thirds of the helix (**Fig. 14**). To block these 2 nerves, one should first retract the helix anteriorly with the thumb of the nondominant hand, then insert the needle behind the inferior aspect of the earlobe. One should aspirate and inject 3 to 4 mL of anesthetic while advancing the needle superiorly, following the curve of the posterior sulcus (**Fig. 15**).[11]

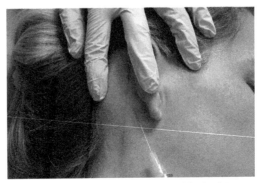

Fig. 15. Greater auricular and lesser occipital nerve block. (*Courtesy of* Alisa Gibson, MD, DMD. University of Maryland School of Medicine, Baltimore, MD.)

SUMMARY

Regional nerve blocks are exceptionally useful in the application of analgesia to wounds of the face. Successful analgesia improves cosmesis, increases patient satisfaction, and reduces discomfort during wound repair.

REFERENCES

1. DeBoard RH, Rondeau DF, Kang CS, et al. Principles of basic wound evaluation and management in the emergency department. Emerg Med Clin North Am 2007;25:23–9.
2. Maurice SC, O'Donnell JJ, Beattie TF. Emergency analgesia in the paediatric population. Part II pharmacological methods of pain relief. Emerg Med J 2002; 19:101–5.
3. Paoli J, Halldin C, Sandberg C. Teaching peripheral nerve blocks for the head and neck area to dermatologists. J Eur Acad Dermatol Venereol 2012;26(8): 1035–7.
4. Nolte J. Cranial nerves and their nuclei. In: Nolte J, editor. The human brain: an introduction to its functional anatomy. 5th edition. Philadelphia: Mosby; 2002. p. 303.
5. Agur AM, Daily AF. Head. In: Grant's atlas of anatomy. 12th edition. Baltimore: Lippincott Williams & Wilkins; 2008.
6. Netter FH. Head and neck. In: Atlas of human anatomy. 4th edition. Philadelphia: Elsevier; 2006.
7. Amsterdam JT, Kilgore KP. Regional anesthesia of the head and neck. In: Roberts JR, Hedges JR, editors. Roberts and Hedges procedural emergency medicine. Philadephia: Saunders Elsevier; 2010. p. 500–12.
8. Zide B, Swift R. How to block and tackle the face. Plast Reconstr Surg 1998; 101(3):840–51.
9. Scheinfeld NS. Inferior alveolar nerve block. 2011. Available at: http://emedicine. medscape.com/article/82622-overview#a01. Accessed April 7, 2012.
10. Malamed SF. Handbook of local anesthesia. 4th edition. St. Louis (MO): Mosby; 1997.
11. Rosh AJ. Ear anesthesia. 2011. Available at: http://emedicine.medscape.com/ article/82698-overview#a15. Accessed April 7, 2012.

Facial Wound Management

Frank Sabatino, MD*, Joshua B. Moskovitz, MD, MPH

KEYWORDS

- Facial wound management • Forehead laceration • Scalp laceration
- Eyelid laceration • Lip laceration • Ear laceration • Auricular hematoma
- Laceration repair

KEY POINTS

- Scalp lacerations: Repair galea using 4-0 nonabsorbable sutures. Repair muscle layer using 4-0 absorbable sutures. Repair skin with 4-0 absorbable sutures or staples.
- Forehead lacerations: The eyebrows must align precisely. Repair muscle layer with 6-0 nonabsorbable sutures. Repair skin with 6-0 nonabsorbable sutures.
- Nose lacerations: Assess the wound for its depth and the anatomy involved.
  - Use 5-0 nonabsorbable sutures that align the rim of the alar margin with skin surrounding the lacerated nare. Leave the suture untied. Place a 5-0 absorbable suture to align the mucosal layer. Place a 5-0 absorbable suture to align the cartilage layer. Tie the original suture.
- Lip lacerations: Place the initial suture to ensure that the vermilion border is aligned precisely. Leave this suture untied. Use an absorbable suture to close the internal mucosal layer. Use a 6-0 nonabsorbable suture to repair the skin layer. Tie the original suture.
- Ear lacerations: Using a scalpel with a #15 blade, make a small incision at the point of maximal fluctuance. Drain the hematoma and irrigate. Place several 4 × 4 gauze pads on the posterior auricle. Place multiple layers of soft gauze on the anterior aspect of the auricle. Place an elastic pressure dressing around the patient's head and tie firmly.

INTRODUCTION

Patients with wounds to the head and face present with significant frequency to the emergency department (ED). Proper technique is vital for optimal wound care to achieve an acceptable cosmetic result and decrease rates of infection.

This article reviews the basic anatomy of the head and face as it relates to wound care. It discusses basic wound management and reviews techniques for repairing cosmetically high-risk areas of the face, particularly the eyes, lips, and ears. Also described are the proper techniques for the management of an auricular hematoma.

Department of Emergency Medicine, North Shore University Hospital, Hofstra North Shore-LIJ School of Medicine, 300 Community Drive, Manhasset, NY 11030, USA
* Corresponding author.
E-mail address: franksabs@gmail.com

Emerg Med Clin N Am 31 (2013) 529–538
http://dx.doi.org/10.1016/j.emc.2013.01.005
0733-8627/13/$ – see front matter Published by Elsevier Inc.

INITIAL WOUND MANAGEMENT

Initial wound care of a head and facial wound is the same as applied to a wound anywhere on the body. The wound should be fully cleansed and examined throughout. All foreign bodies, debris, and dried blood should be removed. The choice of anesthetic and its method of delivery depend on the location of the wound, the mechanism of injury, and the practitioner's comfort level with various techniques, including local administration, regional nerve blocks, and topical anesthetics.[1]

Wound closure can be achieved using sutures, staples, or tissue adhesive. Specific wounds are discussed in the following sections. Suture choice is based on the location and size of the wound (**Table 1**). When sutures are placed on facial skin, they should be positioned 1 to 2 mm from the skin edge and approximately 3 mm apart, which is closer than in other sites on the body. This technique allows better tissue approximation and improved cosmetic outcomes.[1] Suture material is classified in 2 broad groups: nonabsorbable and absorbable. Nonabsorbable sutures need to be removed after placement. For pediatric patients and those with questionable follow-up reliability, absorbable chromic sutures or cat gut can be used for adequate repair of facial skin.[1,2] Staples provide a more rapid alternative for wound closure than sutures.[3] Tissue adhesives also provide a quick and painless alternative to traditional sutures, and can achieve acceptable cosmetic results.[4] This option should be taken into consideration especially in children. The optimal wounds to be repaired with tissue adhesives are small (<3 cm) linear lacerations.[5]

SCALP LACERATIONS

Lacerations on the face and scalp account for roughly 50% of the wounds treated in EDs in the United States.[6,7] Scalp wounds are challenging to address because of the abundant blood flow to the area. Injury in this area is frequently caused by a heavy

Table 1		
Optimal suture material for facial wounds		
Site of Injury	Optimal Suture Size	Optimal Suture Material (Good Alternative Choice)
Cheek, forehead, nose skin	5-0, 6-0	Nylon, prolene (cat gut or chromic for pediatric patients or patients who will not return for removal)
Ear skin	4-0	Nylon (chromic)
Eyelid skin	6-0, 7-0	Nylon (chromic)
Frontalis (forehead) muscle	3-0, 4-0	Vicryl (chromic)
Galea	3-0, 4-0	Vicryl (chromic)
Lip or intraoral mucosa	4-0	Chromic (Vicryl)
Lip muscle	4-0	Vicryl (chromic)
Lip skin	5-0, 6-0	Nylon (chromic)
Nasal mucosa	5-0	Chromic
Scalp skin	3-0, 4-0	Nylon, staples, chromic
Subcutaneous tissue	4-0, 5-0	Vicryl (chromic)

Prolene can be substituted whenever nylon is recommended.
Data from Semer NB. Practical plastic surgery for non-surgeons. Philadelphia: Hanley and Belfus; 2001.

impact, producing irregular deep wounds that complicate optimal cosmesis. The surface area of the head and scalp varies, and visible scars can be readily evident. The consequences of scars can go beyond physical means and may begin to contribute to mental disorders such as depression and posttraumatic stress disorder.[8,9] Scars can also influence patients' rates of unemployment and substance abuse.[9] Because of the potentially significant effects of poor wound repair, the emergency physician (EP) should consider involving consultants in the care of patients with scalp lacerations.[6,10]

The evaluation of a scalp wound is often limited because of excessive bleeding. The area is supplied by a rich vascular network: the arterial supply originates with 3 branches off the external carotid artery and 2 branches off the internal carotid artery.[11] Initial management consists of applying direct pressure and clamping vessels, as necessary.[6,10]

Once hemostasis is obtained, the wound is palpated to examine the depth and condition of the scalp. The scalp anatomy consists of 5 layers: skin, superficial fascia, galea aponeurotica, loose areolar tissue, and pericranium. The examiner should note if there is an obvious depression indicating skull fracture.[6,10]

Anesthesia for scalp lacerations can be provided in multiple ways—topically, locally, or regionally—and the choice depends on the mechanism of injury as well as the practitioner's level of comfort. Topical anesthesia is the least painful of the 3 methods and is sufficient in a considerable number of patients. The advantage of local anesthesia with inclusion of epinephrine is that it can aid in hemostasis and pain control. Regional anesthesia through a supraorbital block will anesthetize an entire side of the forehead as well as the proximal third of the anterior scalp. The regional approach may improve cosmetic outcome by not altering wound margins through subcutaneous infiltration of fluid. Pediatric patients may benefit from sedation.

Irrigation of scalp wounds depends on the mechanism of injury. All traumatic and contaminated wounds should be irrigated to reduce levels of harmful bacteria.[12] However, for a nonbite, noncontaminated wound in a patient who presents within 6 hours, routine irrigation does not alter rates of infection.[13] In prepping for repair of scalp lacerations, shaving will increase the likelihood of infection and therefore is not recommended.[12,13]

Scalp laceration repair should proceed according to the depth of injury.[6] Lacerations to the galea need repair, which should be done with 4-0 nonabsorbable nylon or polypropylene sutures in interrupted or horizontal mattress fashion. This deep suture will improve cosmesis of the final scar and minimize the formation of galeal hematoma. Lacerations involving the muscle layer should be repaired with 4-0 absorbable sutures in simple interrupted fashion. Skin and muscle can be repaired with a single suture through both layers, provided there is no large defect in the muscle layer. The skin can be closed with surgical staples or sutures.[14] When using sutures, 4-0 nylon or rapidly absorbing material should be placed in an interrupted fashion. It is helpful to the practitioner removing the sutures if the color of the suture is different from the patient's hair and if longer tails of sutures are created (**Fig. 1**).[6,15]

After repair of a large or deep laceration, the patient should be discharged with a pressure dressing in place to prevent development of a hematoma.[10]

FOREHEAD LACERATIONS

Repair of forehead lacerations is similar to that of scalp lacerations.[6,10] However, lacerations that involve the muscular layer of the forehead can produce more apparent abnormalities and visual scars when the muscles of facial expression are involved;

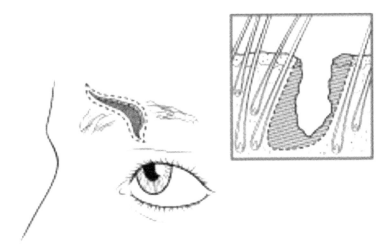

Fig. 1. Do not shave eyebrows. Eyebrows are landmarks for repair and must align perfectly. (*From* Gonzalez del Rey JA, DiGiulio GA. Special anatomical sites. In: Trott A, editor. Wounds and lacerations: emergency care and closure. 3rd edition. Philadelphia: Elsevier Mosby; 2005. p. 161–8; with permission.)

therefore, extreme care should be taken to reapproximate the muscles and to line up the skin tension lines and hair lines exactly to minimize this effect. For deep forehead wounds, 5-0 intradermal absorbable sutures should be used. The skin can be closed with 6-0 nonabsorbable sutures in simple interrupted technique. The epidermal layer of the skin can also be closed with a skin adhesive as long as deeper structures have been repaired and there is minimal tension on the wound.[6,10]

The eyebrows should never be shaved or clipped,[16] because they are important landmarks for the approximation of wound edges. When repairing lacerations involving the eyebrows, it is imperative that hair margins line up precisely.[6,16] Similar to scalp wounds, it is recommended to use a suture color different from the patient's hair color and to leave long tails of sutures to ease the suture-removal process.

EYELID LACERATIONS

Eyelid anatomy consists of 5 layers of tissue, from superficial to deep: skin, subcutaneous tissues, orbicularis oculi, tarsal plate, and conjunctiva.[6,11] The skin of the eyelid is thin and does not provide significant protection to the globe against penetrating objects. The orbicularis oculi is the muscle that controls lid closure. The tarsal plate consists of dense elastic and connective tissue, and contains the meibomian glands and the eyelashes. Nerve supply to the eyelid originates from the temporal and zygomatic branches of the facial nerve.[11]

Wound repair of eyelid lacerations should be initiated only after a thorough eye examination that includes assessment of visual acuity, extraocular muscle performance, examination of the cornea for abrasions and/or foreign bodies, and, most importantly, the potential for globe rupture. Because the eyelids are both functionally and cosmetically important, the EP should consider referring the patient to an ophthalmologist or oculoplastic surgeon. This referral should be automatic for patients with wounds involving the inner surface of the lid, the lid margin (**Fig. 2**), or the lacrimal duct, for injuries associated with ptosis, and for injuries that extend into the tarsal

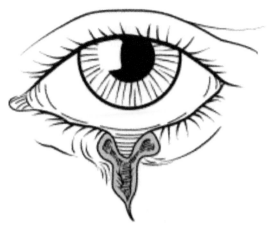

Fig. 2. A vertical intramarginal lid laceration is best left to a consultant to repair. (*From* Gonzalez del Rey JA, DiGiulio GA. Special anatomical sites. In: Trott A, editor. Wounds and lacerations: emergency care and closure. 3rd edition. Philadelphia: Elsevier Mosby; 2005. p. 161–8; with permission.)

plate.[6,16] An injury to the lacrimal duct should be considered in full-thickness eyelid lacerations located within 6 to 8 mm of the medial canthus.[1] Superficial lacerations of the eyelid can be repaired using 6-0 or 7-0 nonabsorbable nylon or polypropylene sutures placed in a simple interrupted fashion (**Fig. 3**).[6,15]

NOSE LACERATIONS

The nose consists of cartilaginous and osseous structures that are separated into halves by the septum. The vital step in evaluating nasal lacerations is assessing the depth and anatomy involved.[17,18]

In some cases, anesthesia can be achieved by inserting cotton swabs or gauze pads soaked with lidocaine and epinephrine into the nasal cavity and then removing them before repair.[6] If this is insufficient, local or regional anesthesia may be used.

Superficial lacerations can be closed with 6-0 nonabsorbable sutures in an interrupted fashion, taking care to preserve any damaged cartilage under the repair of the laceration. Deeper lacerations that involve all tissue layers should be closed as follows[17,18]:

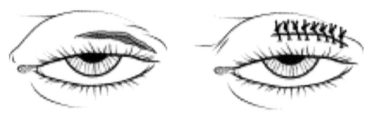

Fig. 3. Extramarginal lacerations to the eyelid can be repaired with a simple row of percutaneous sutures. (*From* Gonzalez del Rey JA, DiGiulio GA. Special anatomical sites. In: Trott A, editor. Wounds and lacerations: emergency care and closure. 3rd edition. Philadelphia: Elsevier Mosby; 2005. p. 161–8; with permission.)

- First, place a 5-0 nonabsorbable suture to align the skin of the alar margin and the skin of the nare, but leave this stitch untied.
- Manipulate the initial stitch with slight traction to align the mucosal and cartilage layers.
- Use 5-0 absorbable suture to secure the mucosal layer.
- If necessary, use a second 5-0 absorbable suture to approximate the cartilage layer.
- Tie the original stitch.
- Reevaluate the intersection between the alar margin and the nare to ensure that the approximation will give the best cosmetic results.[17,18]

Trauma to the nose can result in the formation of a septal hematoma (**Fig. 4**), which requires drainage. Inserting an 18-gauge needle into the hematoma typically will suffice. Alternatively, an incision may be made. Nasal packing should be inserted after drainage, and prophylactic antibiotics must be prescribed (**Fig. 5**).[17,18]

LIP LACERATIONS

The approach to the repair of lip lacerations depends on the structures involved.[6,18–20] The relevant anatomy of the lips consists of 3 surfaces: the skin, the vermilion, and the oral mucosa.[18] The key to proper repair of lip laceration is alignment of the vermilion border.[6,18] Sensation to the upper lip is supplied by the infraorbital nerve, and sensation to the lower lip by the mental nerve.[19,20] Regional anesthesia is convenient for repairing lip lacerations and provides a good opportunity for optimal cosmetic outcome.[1]

The major cosmetic challenge to the repair of lip lacerations is a wound that crosses the vermilion border. When repairing this type of wound, the first stitch must align the edges of the vermilion border exactly (**Fig. 6**). It can be left untied until the remainder of the laceration is repaired.[1,6,15,17]

Intraoral lip lacerations may not need to be sutured, but they do need a full evaluation for foreign bodies such as tooth fragments and food particles,[6,17,18] and should be irrigated before repair. When closure is necessary, absorbable sutures should be used.

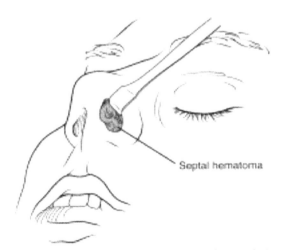

Fig. 4. Septal hematoma in the area of the nasal septum. Failure to drain can lead to septal necrosis and collapse. (*From* Gonzalez del Rey JA, DiGiulio GA. Special anatomical sites. In: Trott A, editor. Wounds and lacerations: emergency care and closure. 3rd edition. Philadelphia: Elsevier Mosby; 2005. p. 161–8; with permission.)

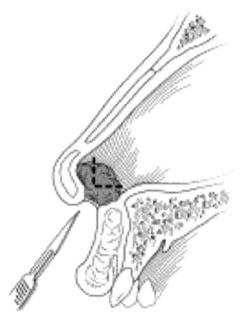

Fig. 5. Technique to drain a septal hematoma. A No. 11 blade is used to create a hockey-stick incision. After drainage, the nose is packed with gauze impregnated with petroleum jelly (Vaseline). (*From* Gonzalez del Rey JA, DiGiulio GA. Special anatomical sites. In: Trott A, editor. Wounds and lacerations: emergency care and closure. 3rd edition. Philadelphia: Elsevier Mosby; 2005. p. 161–8; with permission.)

Through-and-through lacerations should be closed in layers, starting with the mucosal layer, followed by the muscle layer and the orbicularis oris. The muscle layer is closed using an absorbable suture in either a simple interrupted or horizontal mattress fashion. The external mucosa of the lip is then repaired in an interrupted

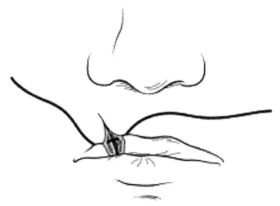

Fig. 6. The major goal when closing any lip laceration is to align the appropriate borders. Initial suture placement and alignment of the vermilion border is shown. When the vermilion border (*line*) is aligned, the remainder of the laceration is closed. (*From* Gonzalez del Rey JA, DiGiulio GA. Special anatomical sites. In: Trott A, editor. Wounds and lacerations: emergency care and closure. 3rd edition. Philadelphia: Elsevier Mosby; 2005. p. 161–8; with permission.)

fashion with 4-0 absorbable sutures; 6-0 nonabsorbable sutures should be used for any portion of the laceration that extends onto the skin (**Fig. 7**).[1,6,15,17]

EAR LACERATIONS

The anatomy of the ear consists of the external ear canal, the auricle, and the lower earlobe. The greater auricular nerve provides sensory innervation, and the blood supply flows from the superficial temporal and posterior auricular arteries. Anesthesia is achieved by performing an auricular block.[6,11]

Superficial wounds to the pinna or helix can be repaired using 6-0 nonabsorbable sutures tied in an interrupted fashion (**Fig. 8**). Through-and-through lacerations that involve the auricle can be repaired by aligning the cartilage with 6-0 nonabsorbable sutures tied in an interrupted fashion. However, most lacerations do not require repair of cartilage, and alignment of the surrounding skin is adequate.[6,21]

Blunt force trauma to the ear can cause tympanic membrane rupture and hematoma formation. A frequent side effect of ear trauma is the formation of an auricular hematoma, also known as cauliflower ear. This type of injury is especially associated with wrestlers, boxers, and mixed martial artists. Treatment is with 1 of 2 techniques. The first option is needle aspiration: using a large-bore needle at the point of maximal fluctuance, the hematoma is aspirated. The second technique uses a scalpel for incision and drainage. A scalpel with a #15 blade is used to make a small incision, less than 5 mm at the point of maximal fluctuation. The hematoma is then drained, followed by irrigation. Regardless of the chosen technique, a pressure dressing is applied to prevent reformation of a second hematoma. After placing several 4 × 4 gauze pads on the posterior aspect of the auricle, multiple layers of soft gauze are placed on the anterior aspect of the auricle. An elastic dressing is placed around the head and

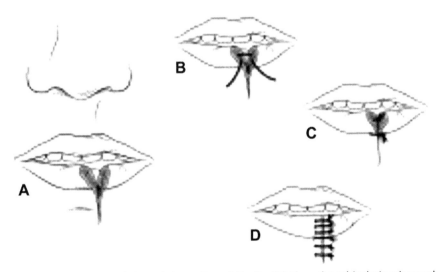

Fig. 7. (*A*) A through-and-through laceration of the lip. (*B*) Close the orbicularis oris muscle with absorbable deep sutures, such as those made of polyglycolic acid. (*C*) When the orbicularis oris muscle is approximated, so is the vermilion border (*line*). (*D*) Close the remainder of the laceration with simple percutaneous monofilament nylon sutures. (*From* Gonzalez del Rey JA, DiGiulio GA. Special anatomical sites. In: Trott A, editor. Wounds and lacerations: emergency care and closure. 3rd edition. Philadelphia: Elsevier Mosby; 2005. p. 161–8; with permission.)

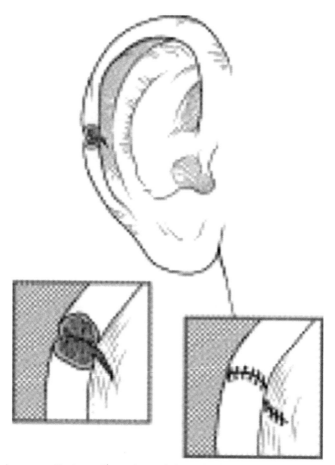

Fig. 8. Simple noncartilaginous lacerations of the ear are closed with either interrupted or running percutaneous skin sutures. (*From* Gonzalez del Rey JA, DiGiulio GA. Special anatomical sites. In: Trott A, editor. Wounds and lacerations: emergency care and closure. 3rd edition. Philadelphia: Elsevier Mosby; 2005. p. 161–8; with permission.)

tied until firm constant pressure is applied. The dressing should remain in place until the patient is reassessed, preferably within 24 hours.[1,6,15,21]

SUMMARY

Facial wound management is of high importance in the ED. Proper techniques must be used to achieve the best results, especially in cosmetically high-risk areas.

The scalp can be repaired in layers. The margins of the eyebrows need to align perfectly. An ophthalmologist or oculoplastic surgeon should be involved immediately for wounds involving the inner surface of the lid, the lid margin, or the lacrimal duct; if the wound is associated with ptosis; and if the wound extends into the tarsal plate. The main objective of the repair of lip lacerations is to ensure that the vermilion border is aligned exactly. Although the incision and drainage of an auricular hematoma can be relatively routine, special consideration must be given to the proper technique of applying a pressure dressing to prevent reaccumulation of the hematoma.

Suboptimal outcomes of any facial wound repair can result in poor wound healing, infection, and significant permanent consequences for patients.

REFERENCES

1. Semer NB. Practical plastic surgery for non-surgeons. Philadelphia: Haley and Belfus; 2001. p. 145–59.
2. Karounis H, Gouin S, Elsman H, et al. A randomized controlled trial comparing long-term cosmetic lacerations repaired with absorbable plain gut versus non-absorbable nylon sutures. Acad Emerg Med 2004;11(7):730–5.
3. Khan AN, Dayan PS, Miller S, et al. Cosmetic outcome of scalp wound closure with staples in the pediatric emergency department: a prospective, randomized trial. Pediatr Emerg Care 2002;18(3):171–3.
4. Sniezek PJ, Walling HW, Debloom JR 3rd, et al. A randomized controlled trial of high-viscosity 2-octyl cyanoacrylate tissue adhesive versus sutures in repairing facial wounds following Mohs micrographic surgery. Dermatol Surg 2007;33(8):966–71.
5. Quinn JV, Drzewiecki A, Li MM, et al. A randomized controlled trail comparing a tissue adhesive with suturing in the repair of pediatric facial lacerations. Ann Emerg Med 1993;22(7):1130–5.
6. Coates WC. Lacerations to the face and scalp. In: Tintinalli JE, Kelen GD, Stapczynski JS, et al, editors. Tintinalli's emergency medicine. 6th edition. New York: McGraw-Hill; 2004. p. 298–304.
7. Hollander JE, Singer AJ, Valentine S, et al. Wound registry: development and validation. Ann Emerg Med 1995;25:675–85.
8. Rankin M, Borah GL. Perceived functional impact of abnormal facial appearance. Plast Reconstr Surg 2003;111(7):2140–6.
9. Levine E, Degutis L, Pruzinsky T, et al. Quality of life and facial trauma: psychological and body image effects. Ann Plast Surg 2005;54(5):502–10.
10. Hollander JE, Singer AJ. Laceration management. Ann Emerg Med 1999;34(3):356–67.
11. Giles WC, Iverson KC, King JD, et al. Incision and drainage followed by mattress suture repair of auricular hematoma. Laryngoscope 2007;117(12):2097–9.
12. Hollander JE, Singer AJ, Valentine SM, et al. Risk factors for infection in patients with traumatic laceration. Acad Emerg Med 2001;8:716–20.
13. Hollander JE, Richman PB, Werblud M, et al. Irrigation in facial and scalp lacerations: does it alter outcome? Ann Emerg Med 1998;31:73–7.
14. Roberts J, Hedges J. Clinical procedures in emergency medicine. 4th edition. Portland (OR): WB Saunders; 2004.
15. Thomsen TW, Barclay DA, Setnik GS. Videos in clinical medicine: basic laceration repair. N Engl J Med 2006;355(17):e18.
16. Howell JM, Morgan JA. Scalp laceration repair without prior hair removal. Am J Emerg Med 1988;6(1):7–10.
17. Brown DJ, Jaffe JE, Henson JK. Advanced laceration management. Emerg Med Clin North Am 2007;25(1):83–99.
18. Trott AT. Wounds and lacerations. 3rd edition. Philadelphia: Mosby; 2005. p. 153–75.
19. Rohen JW. Color atlas of anatomy: a photographic study of human anatomy. 5th edition. Philadelphia: Lippincott; 2005. p. 65–79.
20. Armstrong BD. Lacerations of the mouth. Emerg Med Clin North Am 2000;18(3):471–80.
21. Lavasani L, Leventhal D, Constantinides M, et al. Management of acute soft tissue injury to the auricle. Facial Plast Surg 2010;26(6):445–50.

Management of Facial Fractures

Kim A. Boswell, MD

KEYWORDS

- Frontal sinus fractures • Zygomaticomaxillary complex fractures • LeFort fractures
- Orbital fractures • Naso-orbital ethmoid fractures • Nasal fractures

KEY POINTS

- Facial trauma is commonly seen in the emergency department and presents the emergency physician with potentially life-threatening conditions and associated injuries, including brain and cervical spine injuries.
- Facial fractures are often a part of a constellation of injuries, and the emergency physician should be comfortable recognizing these patterns.
- Frontal fractures require significant force and are often associated with neurologic injury.
- LeFort fractures can be unilateral or bilateral, but all types require involvement of the pterygoid plates.
- Orbital fractures can be subtle and in their presence a full neurologic examination, including evaluation of the cranial nerves, should be performed. Extraocular muscle entrapment is an indication for emergent surgery.
- Surgical intervention of facial fractures is usually not emergent. In those patients who can be safely discharged, good discharge instructions and close follow-up with a facial surgeon are imperative.

The emergency physician must often evaluate patients with facial injuries, including several types of facial fractures. As is typical in our work, we must rapidly determine a patient's stability, placing emergent emphasis on airway, breathing, and circulation. Identifying life-threatening injuries is what we are trained to do; in the setting of facial trauma, these can include bleeding, airway compromise, and associated head or spinal injuries. Most facial fractures are stable injuries that can be addressed with local wound care and appropriate and prompt referral for definitive treatment within the following few days. However, some facial fractures are considered unstable and require more urgent evaluation and treatment. Some fractures are associated with injuries to the cervical spine, globes, dental structures, or lacrimal system. A widely appreciated association is cervical spine injury in conjunction with facial fractures. The incidence of cervical spine fracture has been cited as between 0.3% and 24.0%,[1] but the risk increases with more severe and more numerous facial fractures. It is the emergency physician's responsibility to identify each fracture, understand specific injury patterns, and diagnose commonly associated injuries to the surrounding soft tissue, neurologic structures, or vasculature.

Disclosure: Nothing to disclose.
Surgical Critical Care, Shock Trauma Center, 22 South Greene Street, Baltimore, MD 21201, USA
E-mail address: drkimb@gmail.com

Emerg Med Clin N Am 31 (2013) 539–551
http://dx.doi.org/10.1016/j.emc.2013.01.001
0733-8627/13/$ – see front matter © 2013 Elsevier Inc. All rights reserved.

GENERAL ASSESSMENT

Individuals who present with facial fractures usually have been involved in assaults, motor vehicle crashes, sporting or occupational injuries, or falls. As mentioned previously, initial stabilization of life-threatening injuries is the first priority. Then a general evaluation focusing on the region of the trauma should be performed on every patient with facial injury. Starting with palpation of the facial structure can provide an indication of underlying injury that may not be readily apparent and can elicit instability, as is characteristic of LeFort fractures. Palpation of the cervical spine should be routine practice in the evaluation of patients with facial trauma.

A preliminary visual assessment should be performed in every patient, as well as a full visual acuity, fluorescein/slit-lamp examination in those with injuries to the surrounding structures. If the physician is concerned about globe rupture or laceration, the patient's eye should be covered with a metal shield to prevent *any* pressure from being placed on it until an ophthalmologist can evaluate the patient. Pressure can result in worsening of the injury and permanent vision loss.

Jaw or dental injuries should be evaluated by having patients occlude their teeth. Any malocclusion, difficulty in maintaining a firm bite, or significant pain with jaw opening should raise concern about a mandibular fracture. Intraoral evaluation is essential so that an alveolar ridge or open mandibular fracture is not missed.

A cranial nerve examination should be performed to rule out extraocular muscle entrapment, paresthesias resulting from nerve damage, and impingement.

FRONTAL SINUS FRACTURES

The frontal bone creates the outward appearance of the forehead and is considered part of the skull. For this reason, fractures of the frontal sinus are actually defined as skull fractures.

Anatomy

We are born with a frontal bone but without frontal sinuses. The frontal sinuses begin to develop at the age of 1 or 2 years and are not fully developed to adult size until approximately 12 years of age. In teenagers and adults, the frontal bone is a divided, air-filled structure, pyramidal in shape. It contains the sinus between an anterior and a posterior wall, which are more commonly referred to as "tables." The anterior table is considered the structurally stronger of the two. Inferiorly, the superior orbital rim defines the floor of the sinus. The floor of the frontal sinus composes a large portion of the medial orbital roof. Immediately adjacent and adherent to the posterior table is the dura. A posterior table fracture can be considered an open skull fracture that could allow a cerebrospinal fluid (CSF) leak.

The nasofrontal duct (NFD) is the sole source of drainage for the frontal sinuses and is intimately associated with the frontal bone. It lies against the posteromedial aspect of the frontal sinus floor and is angled in an anterior and inferior direction. It drains into the nasal cavity by way of the uncinate process. Only approximately 15% of the population has a true NFD, and the specific location and course of the NFD are subject to significant individual variability.[2]

Epidemiology

The frontal bone is involved in 5% to 15% of facial fractures and includes fractures that are isolated to either the anterior or posterior table or that involve both of them.[3] The frontal sinus is the strongest bone of the face. Significant force is needed to fracture it, so patients with this injury should be considered at risk for other potentially significant injuries. In fact, concomitant craniofacial injuries are present in approximately 56% to 87% of patients with frontal sinus fracture.[4]

Diagnosis and Management

Frontal bone fractures are most commonly diagnosed with computed tomography (CT). Once diagnosed, several factors determine the need for consultation and surgical intervention. The degree of displacement of the anterior table will affect the cosmetic result once swelling has resolved; therefore, the greater the displacement, the more likely surgical fixation will be necessary. Although the anterior table is the structurally stronger component, the posterior table serves a more protective and functionally important role than its counterpart. Given the proximity of the posterior table to the dura mater and brain tissue, displaced fractures should heighten the physician's concern about possible damage to them. As for the anterior table, the greater the displacement of the posterior table, the more likely is associated injury to underlying structures. Comminution of the posterior table or obvious interruptions in the dura increases the risk for CSF leak. Rhinorrhea from any patient with frontal bone fractures should be considered a CSF leak until proven otherwise. Assessment for the presence of β-2 transferrin is the current "gold standard" to diagnose a CSF leak. Several other bedside tests have been proposed as ways of detecting CSF in body fluids, including glucose testing and the halo test, but none is sensitive or specific.

Frontal bone fractures are rarely an isolated injury, given the force required to induce them. In the rare instance an isolated fracture is present, the patient's disposition depends on the severity of the injury and the presence or absence of associated complications. Patients with an isolated, nondisplaced anterior table fracture with no associated complications can be safely discharged home with close plastic surgery (or facial surgery) follow-up. They should be discharged with nasal and oral decongestants. It is recommended that they undergo repeat imaging to ensure proper healing and prevention of complications at approximately 6 weeks.[5] Patients who have fractures that involve both tables, significant displacement, or comminution or who have associated injuries should be admitted for close evaluation for CSF leak, ophthalmologic evaluation, and potential surgical intervention.[6]

Complications and Associated Injuries

More than half of patients with frontal bone fractures have associated neurologic injuries (**Table 1**).[2] These injuries can vary widely from loss of consciousness to intracranial bleeding. Up to 10% of patients with frontal fractures have subdural or epidural hematomas that require immediate surgical intervention.[7] CT evaluation of the head and cervical spine should be considered essentially routine components of evaluation in patients with frontal bone fractures.

Severe frontal fractures have the ability to extend into the temporal bones and should prompt the emergency physician to evaluate the patient's hearing and facial nerve function. Obtaining temporal bone cuts on CT scan in patients with particularly bad fractures may be beneficial, as true temporal bone involvement requires additional medications, warnings, and follow-up with an otorhinolaryngologist to evaluate for associated hearing loss. Otorrhea in the setting of a temporal bone fracture should also be considered a CSF leak until proven otherwise.

Ocular injuries are not uncommon when frontal sinus fractures involve the supraorbital rim. In fact, up to 25% of people with frontal bone fractures have an ocular injury. In these instances, injury to the globe itself (eg, globe rupture or laceration) or a vision-threatening injury might be present and will need to be evaluated by an ophthalmologist. The most

Table 1
Facial fractures and associated injuries

Fracture Type	Common Associated Injuries Not to Miss
Frontal sinus	Cerebrospinal fluid leak
	Nasofrontal duct involvement/damage
	Ocular injury
	Neurologic injury
Zygomaticomaxillary	Facial paresthesia
	Oribtal apex injury: cranial nerve involvement
LeFort	Dental or alveolar ridge fractures
	Cerebrospinal fluid leaks
	Severe epistaxis
Orbital	Globe rupture or laceration
	Visual field or acuity changes
	Traumatic optic neuropathy
	Optic nerve impingement
	Extraocular muscle entrapment
Nasal	Septal hematoma
	Septal deviation
	Septal mucosal injury
	Epistaxis

commonly associated ocular finding is an afferent papillary defect, which is seen in about 10% of patients with a frontal sinus fracture.[2]

Another structure at risk for injury with frontal sinus fractures is the NFD. This duct is located along the posteromedial floor of the frontal sinus, which composes the roof of the orbit and drains the frontal sinus into the nasal passage, as stated previously. Fracture of the posterior table or floor of the sinus can be associated with interruption, obstruction, or complete disruption of the NFD, which will require surgical repair or obliteration of the sinus cavity to ensure proper drainage to prevent mucocele and mucopyocele formation.[6]

Approximately 6% of patients with frontal sinus fractures (regardless of the presence of CSF leak) will have a course complicated by the development of meningitis. Fractures in the posterior table that involve the dura or are associated with CSF leak brain injury increase the risk of meningitis. The risk is also increased in those who have undergone surgical repair of their posterior table fracture and dura.[8]

The development of complications several years following the original injury is very uncommon. When late complications do emerge, they can be potentially life threatening. This scenario should be considered in the differential diagnosis when assessing patients with a history of frontal sinus fracture. Late complications can include cavernous sinus thrombosis, mucopyocele and mucocele, brain abscess, and encephalitis. Recurrent surgical intervention might be required.

MIDFACE FRACTURES
Zygomaticomaxillary Complex Fractures

Anatomy
The zygomaticomaxillary (ZMC) complex is a quadripod composed of the lateral and inferior orbital rims, the zygomatic arch, and the zygomaticomaxillary buttress. Given that 2 of the 4 "legs" of the quadripod are part of the orbital structure, the ZMC is important in maintaining the integrity of orbital volume and contents. Several buttresses are incorporated in the ZMC: the zygomaticomaxillary buttress, the zygomaticotemporal

buttress, and the zygomaticofrontal buttress. These are points of articulation between facial bones that are common sites of fracture. These articulation points, or sutures, are inherently weak, resulting in an increased likelihood of fracture at these sites. Fracture patterns have been defined differently in many classification schemes. The most widely used is the scheme created by Zingg and colleagues,[9] which divides the fracture patterns into types A, B, and C and contains subtypes depending on the number of components fractured and the severity/displacement of the fractures (**Table 2**). Although many classifications exist, few are truly clinically relevant and are often used more for research and for clarity of physician communication.

Epidemiology

As is common with most facial bone fractures, most ZMC fractures occur as a result of motor vehicle crashes, assaults (via direct blows to the cheek bone), falls, and sporting incidents. Injuries are more common in men than women and occur most often in people between the ages of 20 and 41 years. Alcohol is involved approximately 35% of the time.[10]

Diagnosis and management

Significant swelling, ecchymosis, and pain are the most common presenting complaints and findings in a patient with a ZMC fracture. Several physical signs revealed by examination should heighten the physician's suspicion of a fracture to the ZMC complex. Enophthalmos, or an otherwise malpositioned globe, because of orbital fracture is common, as is subconjunctival hemorrhage. Deformity may be present as palpable emphysema or step-offs over any aspect of the complex, but it is often obscured by the degree of swelling over the cheek or in the periorbital region. The inferior orbital nerve tracks through the orbital floor, so in the setting of a ZMC fracture, evaluation of sensory deficit in the regions of the ipsilateral cheek, inferior eyelid, nose, and upper lip can demonstrate paresthesia or hyperesthesia if the nerve is entrapped or damaged. Documentation of paresthesias by the emergency physician is crucial because 70% to 90% of them are permanent.[11] Diplopia is a common symptom if the extraocular muscle is entrapped. An ocular evaluation is imperative, because almost any ocular or sensory complaint can be justified.

CT is the imaging modality of choice for ZMC fractures, given the variability and combination of fracture patterns that can occur. CT allows the physician to evaluate globe, nerve, and extraocular muscle involvement. Three-dimensional reconstructions can be helpful when evaluating displacement of the fractures in addition to offering surgeons a clearer idea of the severity of the injuries.

Alternatively, some clinicians suggest that plain radiographs, including a Waters, a Caldwell, and an underexposed submental view, can provide sufficient information to make the diagnosis. Given the availability and improved quality of CT scans, they are more reasonable and practical to obtain than plain radiographs.

The structural integrity and prominence of the zygomatic bone make it an important aspect of the facial structure. Fractures that are minimally or nondisplaced and are not

Table 2	
Zingg zygomaticomaxillary fracture types	
Type A	Incomplete fractures • Isolated lateral orbital rim • Isolated inferior orbital rim
Type B	Classic tetrapod fractures or simple malar fractures (noncomminuted)
Type C	Comminuted fractures

comminuted can usually be managed without surgical intervention; however, all fractures of the ZMC complex should be evaluated by a facial surgeon. For ZMC fractures that are comminuted or displaced, open reduction is the treatment of choice, with the goal being to reduce the displacement and restore the facial structure. Additional factors that may lead to surgical repair include involvement of the orbital floor and/or the orbital apex. Fractures of the orbital floor alter the volume within the orbital structure and can be outwardly appreciated as enophthalmos. The orbital apex is the region of the orbit that surrounds the optic nerve and is in close approximation to the internal carotid artery and the cavernous sinus. Fractures in the orbital apex can lead to several other significant injuries, including damage to the internal carotid artery or cavernous sinus or compromise of any of the cranial nerves that run within the cavernous sinus in addition to direct damage to the optic nerve itself. Realignment of a single aspect of a comminuted fracture does not ensure the remainder of the complex is reduced properly. Even slightly misaligned fractures can lead to asymmetry in the face and poor cosmetic results; thus, it is important for the emergency physician to involve a facial surgeon early. It is not uncommon, however, that surgical intervention and repair will be delayed for several days to allow swelling to diminish.

Complications and associated injuries
One associated injury that should induce clinical concern is fracture to the orbital apex with cranial nerve compromise (see **Table 1**). CT scans can demonstrate the involvement of the apex, as well as identify comminuted bone impinging on the optic nerve. In addition to direct compromise of the optic nerve, cranial nerves II, III, IV, V1, and VI all are in close proximity to the apex and can be damaged by fracture to this structure, making a full cranial nerve examination essential in the evaluation of ZMC fractures.[12]

LeFort Fractures

The LeFort fracture classification was named after a French surgeon, Rene LeFort, early in the twentieth century. LeFort studied blunt facial trauma by applying different magnitudes of force and angle to the faces of cadavers. LeFort fractures are usually caused by direct blows to the face and are divided into 3 progressively severe categories, as described later in this article. In real life, fracture patterns are rarely considered "classic" LeFort fractures, but the classification and terminology are still used to describe midface fractures. Each type describes a series of fractures commonly seen in a pattern rather than a single, isolated fracture.

Anatomy
The 3 types of LeFort fractures can occur in any combination and can be unilateral, bilateral, or both. By definition, all types of LeFort fractures involve a fracture of the pterygoid plates. The absence of a pterygoid fracture rules out a LeFort fracture, but the presence of a pterygoid fracture does not specifically imply a LeFort fracture exists. If a pterygoid fracture is noted on CT scan, the emergency physician should have a high index of suspicion for a LeFort-type injury.

LeFort I fractures are horizontal fractures of the maxilla, above the dental structures, and involve the inferior nasal aperture. The fracture extends through the maxilla below the ZMC junction. This constellation of fractures results in a separation the upper jaw from the remainder of the face, sometimes referred to as a "floating palate."

LeFort II fractures involve all of the boney components in a LeFort I, but rather than being a horizontal-type fracture, it is more of a pyramidal shape that extends upward to incorporate a fracture of the zygomaticomaxillary buttress, through the orbital floor and inferior orbital rim into the medial orbital wall and posteriorly into the nasal septum.

As the fracture courses through the maxilla and zygoma, it continues through the upper aspect of the pterygoid plates. The nasal complex and maxilla are divided from the rest of the face.

In LeFort III fractures, the naso-orbital ethmoid complex, zygomas, and maxilla are separated from the cranium. The fracture pattern extends from the nasal bridge downward through the orbit (involving the medial and lateral walls and the floor) and continues through the zygomaticofrontal buttress, thereby including the entire zygomatic arch, causing complete dissociation of the facial structure from the cranial base. For this reason, type III LeFort fractures are also called craniofacial separation or craniofacial dysjunction.

There can be multiple types of LeFort fractures on one side of the face and none on the other, or there can be a variety of types on each side of the face. The presence of one type of LeFort fracture on one side of the face does not indicate there is a LeFort fracture on the other. However, in the setting of facial trauma severe enough to cause a LeFort fracture of any type, the remainder of the boney facial structure should be evaluated for additional fracture patterns, including ZMC and naso-orbital ethmoid fractures.

Diagnosis and treatment

The physical examination findings for each fracture type vary from the others. Physical findings can include a swollen upper lip and a characteristic grating sensation when the hard palate is manipulated, which are commonly seen in type I fractures. Impacted maxillary fractures may not demonstrate mobility, but there may be a grating sensation with attempted movement of the hard palate.

Type II fractures often have more significant deformity and swelling associated with them. Telecanthus (widening of the intercanthal space) is often noted owing to the location of the nasal septum fracture. Subconjunctival hemorrhage and infraorbital ecchymosis can be bilateral, and mobility of the maxilla and hard palate is appreciable.

Type III fractures boast the most significant clinical findings. Significant mobility of the entire facial structure is noted with manipulation. As with the other types, significant facial swelling, deformity, and orbital ecchymosis are almost always present. Associated with severe type II and usually with type III is the "dishface deformity," which is elongation and flattening of the facial structure.

Because fracture types can be found unilaterally, mobility of the face should be tested on both sides as well as in the midline. Sensory deficits in the infraorbital region extending inferiorly to the upper lip can be noted with type II fractures because the fracture pattern involves the inferior orbital rim and floor. The inferior orbital nerve runs along these structures and can easily be affected by fractures. Any deficits should be noted and documented appropriately.

Again, CT scan is the imaging modality that is required to fully and adequately assess the extent of boney and soft tissue injury. Plain films are not sufficient to assess the degree of fracture patterns and displacement. In addition, plain films will not be able to assess associated soft tissue injury.

Involving a facial surgeon early on is always a good idea when assessing a patient with severe facial trauma. The presence of a LeFort fracture is an indication for surgical repair. Lasting cosmetic and functional deficits result from conservative management; the ultimate goals of surgical intervention are to restore the facial projection and the involved sinus cavities and to reestablish proper occlusion of the teeth.

Complications and associated injuries

Epistaxis is commonly associated with LeFort type II and III fractures (see **Table 1**). The location of the bleeding (anterior or posterior) and its severity will drive the decision-making process toward or away from nasal packing. The treatment of choice for severe, life-threatening epistaxis is nasal packing. It is always safer to pack both the posterior and anterior aspects of the nose to obtain hemostasis as rapidly as possible. Life-threatening hemorrhage occurs in 1% to 11% of patients with facial fractures.[13] It is logical to consider catheter-based methods to achieve hemostasis after basic measures, including packing, have been attempted and failed. Published case reports indicate that transcatheter arterial embolization is being used more frequently to treat intractable hemorrhage and has a reported success rate between 87% and 100%.[13,14]

Alveolar and palatal fractures are commonly associated with all types of LeFort fractures and add an element of complexity to the surgical repair. Both types of additional fractures can affect occlusion of the patient's teeth. One of the primary goals of surgical intervention begins with proper occlusion, and proper repair cannot be obtained without good occlusion. If proper occlusion is not obtained, long-term complications with bite are common.

CSF leaks are also frequent complications of primarily type II and type III fractures.[15] CSF rhinorrhea can easily be obscured in the acute setting secondary to epistaxis, but the astute emergency physician should have a high index of suspicion for this complication. As indicated before, assessment for the presence of β-2 transferrin can be requested from the laboratory to confirm the diagnosis of CSF leak. In the presence of a leak, neurosurgical consultation should be obtained early. Antibiotic prophylaxis in the setting of CSF leak remains controversial and should be used at the discretion of the treating neurosurgeon. Treatment with antibiotics should be aimed at broad coverage, which includes the nasal flora.

ORBITAL FRACTURES

Trauma to the eye(s) and periorbital region are common complaints in the emergency department. In fact, approximately 3% of emergency department visits are for traumatic injuries to the eye. A spectrum of injuries and disease processes accompanies these complaints, with some being vision threatening (eg, globe rupture) and others being benign (eg, laceration to the eyebrow). Orbital fractures can be associated injuries that go along with any aspect along the spectrum. Orbital fractures rarely require emergent surgical repair, but additional injuries that do need to be emergently addressed are often present.

Most orbital fractures occur in men between the ages of 21 and 30 years and are the result of assaults and motor vehicle collisions.[16] In the setting of orbital trauma, it is easy to understand why 22% to 29% of orbital fractures are associated with ocular injury.[17]

Anatomy

The structure of the orbit is created by bones of several thicknesses, arranged in a conical shape. Traditionally, the orbit is thought of as a 4-walled structure with a posterior apex. The optic nerve courses through the apex of the cone intracerebrally. The orbital structure is a volume-containing structure that, when fractured, loses its integrity and ability to maintain its volume, often resulting in enophthalmos and compromise to the function of the extraocular muscles.

The frontal bone constitutes part of the superior orbital rim and orbital roof, which contributes the thickness and therefore strength of these 2 structures. The adjoined zygoma and the greater wing of the sphenoid bone make up the lateral wall of the orbit, which is comparatively stronger than its floor and medial wall. The zygoma and maxillary bones create the orbital floor and inferior rim. And, last, the medial wall of the orbit is composed of the ethmoid bone, specifically the very thin-walled lamina papyracea.

There are 2 categories of orbital fractures, pure and unpure, which are also known as blowout fractures and orbital fractures, respectively. Blowout fractures involve only the orbital walls and spare the superior, lateral, and inferior rims. These are usually the result of sudden pressure changes within the orbit, which cause fractures on the thinner and weaker orbital walls, and account for approximately 11% of all orbital fractures.[18] Pure (orbital) fractures can involve any combination of the orbital walls but also involve a fracture of at least 1 of the 3 orbital rims. Orbital fractures are commonly caused by direct forces on the periorbital area. It is not uncommon for orbital fractures to be associated with other patterns, including ZMC, LeFort, and naso-orbital ethmoid fractures. Multiple facial fractures or fracture patterns should alert the emergency physician to the severity of the injury, as they are high-force injuries and can be associated with higher complications, higher rates of concomitant injuries, and a greater likelihood of requiring extensive surgical repair.

Diagnosis and Treatment

Once a patient has been stabilized, facial injuries can be evaluated. Patients with periorbital trauma usually have swelling, ecchymosis, bleeding, and pain. Specifically in orbital trauma, several key areas of evaluation cannot be missed: the globe, pupillary response, extraocular movements, and visual acuity. As previously mentioned, if there is any concern about globe rupture or laceration, the eye should be covered in a fashion that prevents any pressure from being placed on it, and the remainder of the evaluation should be placed on hold until the eye can be assessed by an ophthalmologist. Without indication of globe rupture or laceration, the initial eye examination should start with simple observation of the facial structure. Swelling, obvious deformity, and/or malpositioned globes (eg, appreciable enophthalmos or exophthalmos) can be useful pieces of information. Palpation of the surrounding boney structures can reveal step-offs, representing obvious fracture, and crepitus, representing subcutaneous emphysema, from a fractured medial or inferior orbital wall with communication into the ethmoid or maxillary sinuses, respectively. Visual acuity and fields should be assessed before any direct manipulation of the globe, using a basic Snellen chart. Color perception (including changes in hues) can be difficult to assess, especially in patients who are color blind, but evaluation should be attempted. The presence of binocular diplopia can represent extraocular muscle dysfunction, entrapment, or compression caused by hematoma or swelling. Regardless of the cause of diplopia, it is abnormal and should be considered a result of trauma requiring further evaluation. The globe should be examined for foreign bodies and retained contact lenses (which should be removed). Obvious injuries to the globe, conjunctiva, or lids should be noted. Fluorescein should be used to assess for corneal abrasion or irregularities. Pupillary response, both efferent and afferent, needs a full assessment. Any abnormality, especially an afferent defect, is grounds for ophthalmologic evaluation, as this indicates injury, which may be ongoing, to the optic nerve. If hyphema is present, it should be documented. Extraocular movements should be examined carefully. The inability to demonstrate full range of motion in all directions, thereby using all extraocular muscles, suggests muscle injury or entrapment. Extraocular muscle entrapment is a clinical diagnosis based on restricted range of motion, but CT scan can demonstrate herniated muscle through the fracture line, which can assist in confirming the diagnosis. Patients with entrapped muscle often have associated vagal-type symptoms, including nausea, vomiting, or syncope.

CT scans of the facial bones once again constitute the imaging study of choice. Coronal and sagittal images are beneficial to emergency physicians and facial surgeons in determining the degree of boney displacement and involvement of the apex or in assessing entrapment of the extraocular musculature (**Fig. 1**).

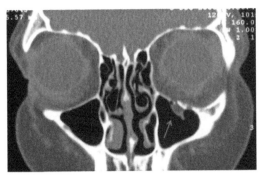

Fig. 1. Blowout fracture with muscle entrapment. Coronal CT scan showing linear trapdoor fracture (*arrow*) of orbital floor. (*From* Gerbino G, Roccia F, Bianchi FA, et al. Surgery for orbital trapdoor fracture. J Oral Maxillofac Surg 2010;68(6):1310–6; with permission.)

Indications for surgical intervention as well as its timing remain controversial. Few orbital fractures mandate emergent intervention. True entrapment of the extraocular musculature within the fracture (including pediatric "trapdoor" fractures [see later in this article]) is an emergent problem, which requires intervention to prevent lasting deficit.[19] Additionally, fractures to the apex of the orbit that result in clinically apparent deficits (eg, traumatic optic neuropathy) or yield radiologic findings that induce concern should undergo urgent operation to reduce pressure or impingement on the optic nerve. Relatively strong indications for surgery include the following: large orbital floor defects (>1 cm), enophthalmos, hypoglobus, or other malpositioning of the globe that persists for weeks following the initial injury.[20] Fractures that do not require surgical intervention are typically managed conservatively. When surgery is indicated, it is usually delayed until swelling and ecchymosis resolve, often in a week to several weeks.

Assuming the patient is stable and has no other injuries causing clinical concern, and after consulting with a facial surgeon, it is often acceptable to discharge patients home to follow up as an outpatient for possible definitive treatment. Patients should be discharged with proper pain management. If fractures extend into the sinuses, the patient should be sent home with "sinus precautions," which include no nose blowing or sneezing with the mouth open.

Complications and Associated Injuries

Traumatic optic neuropathy is the loss of vision, visual fields, or color perception in the setting of periocular trauma and is an indication of direct optic nerve trauma (see **Table 1**). Any change in perception of color or vision loss should be a sign of great concern to the emergency physician, as vision loss can, and often does, become permanent.

Extraocular muscle that is entrapped can easily become ischemic. Prolonged ischemia can lead to muscle damage and long-term impairment in mobility. A "trapdoor" fracture, described within the pediatric population, is a fracture of the orbital floor, in which the bony fragment forms a greenstick fracture after initial displacement, entrapping the inferior rectus muscle. These fractures are often difficult to diagnose, as the orbital volume is maintained and the only symptom may be restriction of ocular movement.

NASAL FRACTURES

The nasal bone is the most commonly broken bone of the face, likely because of its prominence.[21] Like other facial fractures, nasal fractures are usually the result of motor vehicle collisions, assaults, sports incidents, or falls, and often present with swelling, pain, and ecchymosis.

Anatomy

The nasal bone is a pyramidal structure composed of 2 thin bones that become progressively thinner the more distally they project. The most distal aspect and the tip of the nose are composed of cartilage, which is relatively resistant to injury. The more proximal aspect of the nasal bone is thicker and adjoins to the ethmoid bone and the maxilla. The more proximal nasal fractures can extend into the maxilla and ethmoid bone, creating a naso-orbital ethmoid fracture, as previously described.

Diagnosis and Treatment

Nasal fractures can be isolated injuries, or they can be a single fracture among other facial injuries. Patients often have swelling, bruising, epistaxis, infraorbital ecchymosis, and pain. There often is a noticeable deformity to the nasal bridge, but swelling some-times precludes the ability to appreciate it. The physical evaluation of a patient with a suspected nasal bone fracture should include an external examination as well as an internal examination. The external examination should focus on palpation of the nasal bridge for deformities or tenderness in addition to the presence of possible sensory deficits that may indicate additional facial fracture or injury. A properly performed internal examination involves a nasal speculum or otoscope, proper analgesia/anes-thetic, and an inhaled vasoconstrictor. The patient's nasal passages should be anes-thetized with topical lidocaine (4%), and an aerosolized vasoconstrictor should be used to help stop oozing and prevent bleeding during the examination. The examination should focus on the septum, looking for deviation, mucosal injury, and/or hematoma.

When an isolated nasal fracture is suspected, plain radiographs are adequate for diagnosis. The presence of additional facial injuries or other findings that raise concern should encourage the emergency physician to pursue more detailed imaging in the form of a CT scan. The CT scan will properly identify concomitant fractures or soft tissue injuries in addition to the nasal fracture.

A simple nasal bone fracture can be easily treated with ice for swelling, pain control, and time. Comminuted or open fractures require more consideration regarding proper treatment. Patients who present immediately after injury often have not developed substantial swelling, which provides the best window of opportunity to assess the deformity and perform a closed reduction of the fracture. Once swelling develops, deformities are obscured, so waiting several days to a week for the swelling and pain to dissipate is a reasonable treatment plan. In these instances and barring addi-tional injuries preventing discharge, patients should be sent home with pain medica-tions, sinus precautions, and antibiotics if they have open wounds. As with any degree of swelling, elevation and ice are recommended. Referral to a facial surgeon for follow-up within 1 week for evaluation and definitive treatment is appropriate.[22]

Complications and Associated Injuries

Several physical examination findings, even in a patient with an isolated nasal bone fracture, should not be missed by the emergency physician (see **Table 1**). Septal hema-tomas are easy to diagnose and treat. Appropriate treatment can prevent complica-tions, such as septal hematoma infection and/or abscess or necrosis of the septal cartilage with formation of a septal perforation. Straightforward incision and drainage or clot removal from the hematoma with subsequent anterior nasal packing to prevent reaccumulation of the hematoma can prevent these complications from occurring.

Epistaxis is an obvious and frequent complication of nasal fractures. Generally speaking, hemostasis has usually occurred by the time the patient presents to the emergency department, but epistaxis can continue, thus requiring physician intervention. Anterior bleeding from Kiesselbach plexus is common and generally easy to control. Posterior nasal hemorrhage usually originates from the anterior ethmoidal and sphenopalatine arteries and can be more difficult to control. Occasionally, placement of packing (anterior or posterior, depending on the location of the hemorrhage) is required to stop the bleeding. Patients who are discharged with nasal packing in place, for any reason, should be given a prescription for antibiotics that cover gram-positive organisms to prevent infection in addition to strict follow-up instructions for packing removal and further treatment.

Open nasal bone fractures are not uncommon and need additional attention to ensure proper follow-up and prevention of complications. As for all nasal fractures, a thorough physical examination of the nose should be performed and any lacerations should be well irrigated (especially if the injury was caused by a contaminated or soiled object) and sutured closed. Any laceration internally or externally near the site of the fracture should be considered an open fracture, so prophylactic antibiotics should be prescribed.

Copious amounts of clear nasal secretions in a patient with nasal trauma or fracture should prompt the emergency physician to be concerned about a CSF leak. Most CSF leaks can be managed conservatively and resolve spontaneously, but leaks that persist beyond 10 to 14 days should be assessed for possible repair of the dural tear causing the leak.

SUMMARY

Facial trauma is a common complaint in the emergency department. Interventions can range from simply diagnosing a fracture and providing referral, to very complex management of severe fractures requiring stabilization of the airway, hemostasis of active bleeding, and proper evaluation and management of many aspects of trauma. It is vital that emergency physicians recognize associated injuries, including those affecting the brain and cervical spine, as common associations in facial trauma.

The emergency physician must always maintain a high degree of suspicion and should evaluate all complaints of facial trauma thoroughly, because a missed injury can threaten life or vision. A methodical and organized examination is paramount for patient safety and the physician's documentation of the evaluation.

CT scans are the most efficient and comprehensive way to evaluate facial trauma and fractures and should be used liberally in patients with any concern for soft tissue or boney injury and especially in those who are unable to provide a reliable examination. CT scans of the head and cervical spine can be life-saving. Many injuries are obscured by swelling or ecchymosis. It is always safer to consult a facial surgeon in the setting of uncertainty. In patients who are safe for discharge, it is the responsibility of the emergency physician to provide clear instructions regarding close follow-up.

REFERENCES

1. Lynham AJ, Hirst JP, Cosson JA, et al. Emergency department management of maxillofacial trauma. Emerg Med Australas 2004;16:7–12.
2. Manolidis S, Hollier LH Jr. Management of frontal sinus fractures. Plast Reconstr Surg 2007;120(Suppl 2):32S–48S.
3. Metzinger SE, Guerra AB, Garcia RE. Frontal sinus fractures: management guidelines. Facial Plast Surg 2005;21(3):199–206.

4. Fraioli RE, Branstetter BF 4th, Deleviannis FW. Facial fractures: beyond LeFort. Otolaryngol Clin North Am 2008;41:51–76.
5. Tiwari P, Higuera S, Thornton J, et al. The management of frontal sinus fractures. J Oral Maxillofac Surg 2005;63:1354–60.
6. Kalavrezos N. Current trends in the management of frontal sinus fractures. Injury 2004;35:340–6.
7. Gerbino G, Roccia F, Benech A, et al. Analysis of 158 frontal sinus fractures: current surgical management and complications. J Craniomaxillofac Surg 2000;28:133–9.
8. Wallis A, Donald PJ. Frontal sinus fractures: a review of 72 cases. Laryngoscope 1988;98:593–8.
9. Zingg M, Laedrach K, Chen J, et al. Classification and treatment of zygomatic fractures: a review of 1,025 cases. J Oral Maxillofac Surg 1992;50:778–90.
10. Bogusiak K, Arkuszewski P. Characteristics and epidemiology of zygomatico-maxillary complex fractures. J Craniofac Surg 2010;21(4):1018–23.
11. Ceallaigh PO, Ekanaykaee K, Beirne CJ, et al. Diagnosis and management of common maxillofacial injuries in the emergency department. Part 4: orbital floor and midface fractures. Emerg Med J 2007;24:292–3.
12. Linnau KF, Hallam DK, Lomoschitz FM, et al. Orbital apex injury: trauma at the junction between the face and the cranium. Eur J Radiol 2003;48(1):5–16.
13. Wu S, Chen RJ, Lee KW, et al. Angioembolization as an effective alternative for hemostasis in intractable life-threatening maxillofacial trauma hemorrhage: case study. Am J Emerg Med 2007;25:988.e1–5.
14. Liu WH, Chen YH, Hsieh CT, et al. Transarterial embolization in the management of life-threatening hemorrhage after maxillofacial trauma: a case report and review of the literature. Am J Emerg Med 2008;26:516.e3–5.
15. Ceallaigh PO, Ekanaykaee K, Beirne CJ, et al. Diagnosis and management of common maxillofacial injuries in the emergency department. Part 3: orbitozygo-matic complex and zygomatic arch fractures. Emerg Med J 2007;24:120–2.
16. Fonseca RJ. Oral and maxillofacial trauma. St Louis (MO): Elsevier Saunders; 2005.
17. Kraus JF, Rice TM, Peek-Asa C, et al. Facial trauma and the risk of intracranial injury in motorcycle riders. Ann Emerg Med 2003;41:18–26.
18. He D, Blomquist PH, Ellis E 3rd. Association between ocular injuries and internal orbital fractures. J Oral Maxillofac Surg 2007;65(4):713–20.
19. Cole P, Boyd V, Banerji S, et al. Comprehensive management of orbital fractures. Plast Reconstr Surg 2007;120(Suppl 2):57S–63S.
20. Rinna C, Ungari C, Saltarel A, et al. Orbital floor restoration. J Craniofac Surg 2005;16:968–72.
21. Hwang K, You SH, Lee HS. Outcome analysis of sports-related multiple facial fractures. J Craniofac Surg 2009;20:825–9.
22. Mondin V, Rinaldo A, Ferlito A. Management of nasal bone fractures. Am J Otolaryngol 2005;26:181–5.

Mandible Fractures and Dental Trauma

John M. Murray, MD

KEYWORDS

- Dental trauma • Dentoalveolar traumatic injury • Mandible fracture
- Emergency management

KEY POINTS

- Every emergency department should have available basic materials to care for tooth avulsions, luxations, and fractures.
- Proper handling and early replacement of avulsed permanent teeth is essential to long-term retention and good outcome.
- Do not let avulsed teeth dry out. Place in Hanks balanced salt solution or milk at the earliest opportunity.
- Prescribe antibiotics with coverage of oral flora in the case of replaced avulsed teeth. Antibiotic coverage is not suggested for luxation injuries or crown fractures.
- Use computed tomography scan for suspected mandible fractures that are not apparent on plain film radiographs.
- Antibiotics with coverage of oral flora are suggested for open mandible fractures (gingival bleeding or laceration).

INTRODUCTION

Traumatic injury to the teeth and their surrounding, supporting structures is a common occurrence. Various surveys indicate that up to 25% to 50% of the population in certain communities report having sustained such an injury.[1] Association of dentoalveolar traumatic injury (DTI) with other trauma and the inability to access immediate care by a dentist for isolated dental trauma leads many to seek care for these injuries in the emergency department (ED). Estimates are that 3 million emergency room (ER) visits for dental-related complaints occurred in the United States between 1997 and 2000.[2] Recent data indicate that these numbers have continue to grow, with more than 830,000 visits in 2009 alone, an increase of 16% compared with 2006 estimates.[3]

Department of Emergency Medicine, Miles Memorial Hospital, Lincoln County Health, 35 Miles Street, Damariscotta, ME 04543, USA
E-mail address: john.murray@lchcare.org

Emerg Med Clin N Am 31 (2013) 553–573
http://dx.doi.org/10.1016/j.emc.2013.02.002
0733-8627/13/$ – see front matter © 2013 Elsevier Inc. All rights reserved.

DTI most commonly involves the anterior teeth because of their exposed location. The frequency of DTIs is inversely related to patient age, with the greatest incidence occurring in children between 2 and 3 years old, related to falls as new motor skills are developing.[4] The most frequently cited causes of injury to the permanent dentition include falls, motor vehicle accidents, interpersonal violence, and sports-related mishaps, with the relative contribution of each varying among different age groups and locations studied.

Mandible fracture may be found in association with injury or displacement of the teeth or may occur in isolation. The mandible is among the most frequently fractured facial bones, second only to nasal bone fracture in the pediatric population.[5] Common causes of injury include bicycle accidents, motor vehicle collisions, and falls in the young whereas older age groups sustain fractures mostly because of motor vehicle collisions, assaults, and falls.

ED care of such injuries should be seen as temporizing until such time as more definitive dental care can be provided. The timely application of initial care, which is within the scope of practice of emergency medicine providers with some basic equipment and easily mastered skills, can have a significant effect on limiting secondary complications and greatly increase the chance of a positive outcome in these injuries.

Anatomy Review

A basic understanding of dental anatomy is required for proper diagnosis of injuries and planning of initial care and can aid in the description of injury to dental consultants. In addition, the progression from primary (baby teeth or deciduous teeth) to adult (secondary teeth) dentition must be taken into account when formulating treatment plans in some cases.

Adult teeth are 32 in number, arranged in 4 symmetric groups in the right and left maxilla (upper teeth) and right and left mandible (lower teeth). From midline to the back of the mouth there are 1 central incisor, 1 lateral incisor, 1 canine (eye tooth), 2 premolars (bicuspids) and 3 molars (with the most posterior being the wisdom tooth).

Primary teeth number only 20, with each group consisting of 1 central incisor, 1 lateral incisor, 1 canine (eye tooth), and 2 molars.

The most common system of dental nomenclature used in the United States is the Universal Numbering System. Recommended for use by the American Dental Association in 1968, the secondary teeth are numbered starting with the right upper third molar being number 1 and progressing from right to left sequentially across the maxilla to the left upper third molar as number 16. Numbering then continues on the same side of the mouth with the left lower third molar being designated number 17 and then progressing sequentially from left to right across the mandible to number 32 at the right lower third molar. The primary teeth are designated by capital letters starting with A for the right upper second molar and proceeding in a similar fashion across the maxilla and back across the mandible to end with T at the right lower second molar. Several other systems of nomenclature exist and none of them are intuitive if not used frequently. It is therefore suggested that a more simple method of designating the involved teeth based on the location and type of tooth be used in describing injuries and in discussion with consultants (eg, right upper central incisor, left lower canine tooth).

The structure of each tooth consists of the crown or visible portion above the gingiva and the root portion anchored in the alveolar bone. The crown is composed of 3 distinct layers: the enamel, the dentin, and the pulp. Enamel, which is purported to be the hardest substance in the human body, provides the external covering layer of the crown of the tooth. White and pearly in appearance, it provides the surface for mastication and protects the remainder of the tooth from exposure to intraoral contents. Once injured, enamel has no native regenerative capacity.[3] Dentin forms the bulk of the tooth structure and is composed of a porous, microtubular structure. It is more yellow in color and less reflective than enamel. Dentin is produced by the pulp of the tooth in a process that can be stimulated by trauma as long as the pulp remains healthy. Once exposed, the more permeable nature of dentin allows entry of materials likely to cause inflammation and infection to the underlying pulp cavity if proper care is not promptly undertaken. The central pulp consists of a complex of odontoblasts (cells that produce dentin) and fibroblasts in an extracellular matrix and also contains the neurovascular supply to the tooth. Although smaller in volume, it performs the critical role of carrying nutrients to supply the remainder of the tooth. Direct injury or secondary contamination can result in pulp necrosis, one of the major factors leading to poor outcome after dental trauma. Permanent teeth retain some ability to regenerate injured pulp tissue. This capacity is especially retained in teeth that have not yet fully matured as indicated by the continued presence of a visible opening at the tooth apex.[6] Examining avulsed teeth for the presence of this apical opening and documenting its presence may assist follow-up dental care providers in choosing treatment options and predicting long-term viability.

The teeth are anchored in the maxilla or mandible within the alveolar bone. This attachment structure or periodontium is composed of the gingival structures and the periodontal subunit. The free gingiva forms the cuff of tissue around the base of the crown and can sustain laceration with or without the tooth being displaced. Bleeding within the gingival sulcus, the space between the gingival cuff and the crown surface, can indicate injury to the attachment apparatus even in teeth that do not appear to be loosened or displaced.

The outermost layer of the tooth's root is called the cementum, and is attached to the socket in the alveolar bone by the periodontal ligament (PDL). This collagen-based ligament is sensitive to injury when traumatized and its maintenance and survival are critical to the long-term outcome of injured teeth. Damage to the PDL and cementum can result in fusion or resorption of the tooth root, the second major complication associated with poor outcomes after dental trauma.

PRIMARY AND SECONDARY TEETH

The initial approach to the treatment of many traumatic dental injuries depends on whether the injured tooth is part of the primary or permanent dentition. This distinction is especially important when deciding to replace teeth that have been displaced from the socket.

The age at which primary teeth are lost and secondary tooth eruption occurs can be used as an approximate guide in this determination; however, variability does occur (**Table 1**).[7] Obtaining this history from the family offers another viable option.

The developing germinal bud of the permanent tooth lies deep to and in an intraoral (lingual) direction from the primary tooth root structure. Traumatic injury to primary teeth can have a significant impact on subsequent development of the permanent dentition. Associated injury to the secondary tooth bud can lead to arrested or abnormal development. Ankylosis of the primary tooth root or alteration in the dental arch caused by premature tooth loss may interfere with permanent tooth eruption. Given these concerns, appropriate follow-up with a dental provider should be encouraged. Decisions in the ED should be limited to not attempting to reimplant avulsed primary teeth as well as consideration of early removal of severely extruded and loosened primary teeth.

Table 1			
Primary and permanent tooth development by age			
Primary Tooth Age at Eruption (mo)	Primary Tooth Age Shed (y)	Upper Tooth	Permanent Tooth Age at Eruption (y)
8–12	6–7	Central incisor	7
9–13	7–8	Lateral incisor	8
16–22	10–12	Canine	11–12
		First premolar	10
13–19	9–11	First molar	6
25–33	10–12	Second molar	12–13
		Third molar	7–21
Primary Tooth Age at Eruption (mo)	Primary Tooth Age Shed (y)	Lower Tooth	Permanent Tooth Age at Eruption (y)
6–10	6–7	Central incisor	6–7
10–16	7–8	Lateral incisor	8
17–23	9–12	Canine	9–10
		First premolar	10–11
		Second premolar	11–12
14–18	9–11	First molar	6
23–31	10–12	Second molar	11–13
		Third molar	7–21

Data from American Dental Association. Available at: http://www.ada.org. Accessed September 21, 2011.

EVALUATION PRINCIPLES

As in any case of traumatic injury, a systematic, initial evaluation and treatment of injuries that represent a threat to life or function should be carried out as appropriate. Although DTI is, in itself, not life threatening, the effect of resultant bleeding, anatomic derangement, and possible pharyngeal foreign body needs to be considered.

Instability caused by fracture of the anterior mandible, especially when bilateral, may create a tendency to prolapse of the oral soft tissues causing airway obstruction.[8] Altered anatomy caused by injured mandibular or maxillary structures may make manual airway clearing maneuvers and bag valve mask ventilation difficult. Soft tissue swelling of the tongue or floor of the mouth from associated soft tissue or vascular injury may expand rapidly, necessitating early airway intervention. Localized bleeding may be temporized, if time allows, with local injection of anesthetics containing epinephrine. Fractures of the condyles or angle of the mandible may result in a physical impediment to mouth opening during attempted airway visualization that may not be fully overcome even by neuromuscular blockade.[2bb]

While initial evaluation is being carried out, consideration should be given to appropriate storage of any avulsed teeth. As discussed later, this can enhance the likelihood of successful replantation when the clinical situation allows.

History

Specific relevant points should be sought and recorded as part of the standard history-taking process. Mechanism and time since injury should be recorded as well as details regarding the handling of any lost teeth or tooth fragments. Specifics about the way an avulsed tooth was cleansed, any solution that was used to store the tooth en route to the hospital, and time before placement in transport media all dictate initial management strategy. They also are important for the prognosis of survival of the tooth over time and assist in planning long-term management strategies by dentists in follow-up.

Asking the patient about a subjective change in the alignment of the teeth or a change in occlusion can provide a clue to a change in tooth alignment or imply a mandibular fracture.

Whether the injured tooth is part of the primary or secondary dentition can often be determined by questioning the patient or a parent. Past history of bleeding disorders or the use of any medications that affect platelet function or the coagulation cascade should be sought. History of cardiac valve disorders, indwelling hardware, or other factors that would prompt consideration of antibiotics after dental work as well as tetanus status should also be considered.

Evaluation of the teeth should start with a careful inspection for chipped as well as any missing or malaligned teeth. Asking the patient or parent to confirm that any findings are a change from previous baseline can help to identify acute injury. Looking for any blood in the gingival sulcus can be a clue to injury as well. The teeth can then be palpated with a gloved finger or percussed with a tongue blade to assess for tenderness and mobility. Sensitivity of the tooth to cold water or to forced air can help to determine the classification of tooth fractures, as described later. Forced air testing can be performed in the ED without specialized equipment, instead making use of suction tubing or oxygen supply tubing attached to commonly available compressed air or oxygen sources.

Associated lacerations or other soft tissue injuries should be examined to ensure that any lost teeth or fragments are not embedded in the wound. Gingival laceration on the mandibular surface may suggest an open fracture.

Palpate the mandible for tenderness or step-off including the temporomandibular joints (TMJs) to assess for possible fracture. Observation for asymmetry with mouth opening or an inability to fully open may also indicate underlying fracture. Palpation of the maxilla also screens for possible fracture of the supporting structures for the upper teeth.

TOOTH AVULSION

Total loss or avulsion of a tooth, also referred to as complete luxation, represents one of the most impressive dental injuries and is a dental emergency. Proper initial care both in the prehospital and ED setting is critical to the long-term prognosis of the involved tooth. Proper handling of the avulsed tooth and timely reimplantation are critical to avoid the 2 major complications that limit long-term survival of the tooth: pulpal infection and attachment apparatus damage.

Avulsions most frequently involve the maxillary central incisors and represent up to 3% of DTIs.[9] These injures frequently involve a coexistent fracture of the underlying alveolar bone, although this has little practical impact on the initial ED management.

Initial management decisions depend first on determining whether the involved tooth is part of the primary or permanent dentition. Primary teeth should not be reimplanted because of the risk of damage to, and subsequent abnormal development of, the underlying permanent tooth bud. Although the classification of the avulsed tooth can be roughly determined by the age of the patient, obtaining a dental history from the patient or family member is the surest way to make this determination. A panorex will reveal the tooth buds of the permanent teeth if the lost tooth was a primary tooth.

Prehospital Actions

If an avulsed permanent tooth can be located after a traumatic avulsion, optimal outcome is best served by immediate reimplantation at the scene if possible.

The avulsed tooth should be handled by the crown with no contact with the root portion to avoid further damage to the adherent PDL tissue. If visible contamination is evident, a gentle rinse with 0.9% saline solution, if available, or tap water is recommended. At no time should the root of the tooth be physically rubbed or scraped to remove perceived debris. The tooth should then be reinserted gently into the socket. The tooth ideally should be placed in its normal position, but determining the labial from the lingual surface is sometimes difficult. The important thing is to make sure that the root is in contact with the socket. The patient should then be instructed to bite down on a piece of gauze or other clean material to hold the tooth in place while being transported to the ED or a dental professional.

In some cases, personnel at the scene may not able to reinsert the tooth in the socket because of competing treatment priorities or other factors. Concern that the patient may be a risk for aspiration of a tooth that cannot reliably be held in place, or a lack of patient cooperation because of age, altered mental status, or other factors, may play a role. In these cases, proper treatment of the tooth during timely transportation to an appropriate treatment facility can enhance chances for successful reimplantation. Limiting ongoing damage to the PDL cells from drying is critical to maintaining viability until reimplantation can occur.

Numerous studies have shown that Hanks balanced salt solution (HBSS) may be the best medium for the transport and storage of avulsed teeth, and it is currently recommended by the American Association of Endodontics.[10] Readily available in some commercial products, this solution has been shown to maintain PDL cell viability for more than 24 hours and its use is thought to improve the likelihood of retention of the reimplanted tooth. Commercially available kits containing HBSS solution along with a container designed to minimize ongoing trauma to the root are marketed as the Save-a-Tooth system (Phoenix-Lazarus Inc, Pottstown, PA) and EMT Tooth Saver (Biochrom AG, Berlin, Germany). If such a product is unavailable, milk, because of its pH and osmolarity, has been shown to provide suitable conditions for PDL cell preservation for up to 3 hours[10] and represents a readily available alternative. Recent studies have suggested that milk may sustain PDL viability for even longer than is currently stated in the literature. One recent article using an in-vitro model of PDL cell survival showed good viability of PDL cells in milk for up to 48 hours at room temperature and concluded that milk outperformed HBSS in this regard.[11]

In the absence of either of these choices, the tooth can be transported in the patient's own saliva collected in a clean container or in 0.9% saline, if available. Both saline and saliva have been shown to maintain PDL viability for up to 2 hours.

Because of its low osmolarity, water has been shown to result in PDL cell disruption and decreased viability and should be used as a last resort.[12] The practice of transporting the avulsed tooth intraorally under the tongue or in the buccal recess (inside the cheek) is to be discouraged. There is a risk of aspiration of the tooth as well as a risk of friction causing physical damage to remaining tissue adherent to the root.

If the tooth is initially stored in a less optimal solution it should be transferred to a more physiologic medium as soon as one becomes available. This transfer may occur with Emergency Medical Services arrival if they carry an HBSS-like tooth preservation product or on arrival to the ER while further evaluation occurs and the patient is prepared for reimplantation.

ED Actions

After evaluation for and treatment of more life-threatening traumatic injuries, ED personnel should be comfortable with reimplantation of avulsed permanent teeth. While other evaluation and treatment occur and while preparation is made for reimplantation, any avulsed teeth transported with the patient should be placed in the best storage medium available, ideally HBSS.

Relevant history should include ascertaining whether the involved tooth is part of the primary or permanent dentition, as described earlier. Along with standard elements of history taking, additional information should include an estimate of the extraoral dry time and the time from tooth loss until it was placed in some form of transport solution. Available details of how the tooth was handled before ED arrival and what medium was used for tooth storage should be recorded.

If not located at the scene, an evaluation for other possible locations of the missing tooth is required. One possibility includes impaction into the underlying alveolar bone, which may be determined by careful examination and may require radiographs of the maxilla or mandibular area. The possibility that a missing tooth or fragment may be embedded in any coexisting soft tissues should be considered. Careful examination of any wounds by visualization and palpation should be performed with radiographic examination ordered as needed. In addition, the possibility that the missing tooth was aspirated into the tracheobronchial tree or was swallowed may require radiographs that include the chest and upper abdomen. Teeth or tooth fragments located below the level of the diaphragm can be treated with serial observation for passage through the gastrointestinal tract. Endoscopic or bronchoscopic removal of those located in the pulmonary tree or in the esophagus is recommended.

An avulsed tooth that has been properly reimplanted in the prehospital setting and that is in good position can simply be left in place and splinted as described later. If the reimplanted tooth is malpositioned, most commonly a continued partial extrusion, repositioning may require removal and more thorough preparation of the socket.

If the tooth has not been reimplanted before arrival in the ED, preparation of the socket needs to take place.

Obtaining local or regional anesthesia of the involved maxillary or mandibular region using the appropriate dental block makes the patient more comfortable and cooperative during socket preparation and tooth insertion. Options include supraperiosteal injection or other regional dental blocks.[13]

Examination of the socket and surrounding teeth should occur to determine whether there has been any collapse of the socket wall or associated alveolar bone fracture. Adjacent teeth that are loose or misplaced may indicate an alveolar bone fracture. Although dental radiographs or panorex-type films may be helpful in detecting any fracture of the boney support structure commonly available facial radiographs may lack the detail necessary to assess the area well. However, exact details of any alveolar fracture are not critical to emergent care of avulsed or luxated teeth and obtaining radiographs should not delay other care.

Should loosening, displacement, or suspected alveolar fracture be present, the involved teeth should be repositioned to their normal anatomic position (after adequate anesthesia is provided). After reinserting the avulsed tooth, splinting should be performed with a wide enough arc to anchor all of the involved dentition to stable structures.

The socket should be gently irrigated with normal saline using a syringe and Angiocath or blunt-tipped needle. Once cleared of any retained clot, if inspection reveals an inward collapse of the socket wall gentle pressure with a blunt instrument such as a dental mirror handle is recommended to create space to reinsert the tooth root.

The tooth should be handled in much the same way as described earlier. The tooth should be handled by the crown and stored in HBSS, milk, or normal saline (in order of preference) while preparations and other care and evaluation are rendered. Before reimplantation, the root should be gently rinsed of any obvious debris with a low-pressure stream of normal saline.

Recent dental literature suggests that the prognosis and optimal later treatment strategies may differ based on the maturity of the reimplanted tooth.[14] The base of each dental root or apex remains open with a size greater than 1 mm while permanent teeth are maturing. Once the apex is closed (less than 1 mm), the tooth is considered mature. The presence of an adequately open root apex may allow revascularization of the tooth. Because this cannot be determined in individual cases by patient age alone, examination of the root apex and noting the appearance and size of the apical foramen may be helpful to later planning and prognostication from a follow-up dental provider.

Some recent guidelines, citing evidence from animal studies, recommend exposure of the avulsed tooth to topical antibiotics before reimplantation of open apex (immature) teeth, which is performed by soaking the avulsed tooth in a doxycycline solution (1 mg of doxycycline in 20 mL of normal saline or HBSS) for 5 minutes before reimplantation. Thought to act through a reduced bacterial contamination of the remaining PDL and pulpal tissues, improved rates of revascularization as well as decreasing root resorption have been seen in experimental study.[15]

Once the tooth and socket have been thus prepared, the tooth should be gently inserted into the socket. The tooth should then be splinted in place. Dental providers create flexible splints that allow a physiologic degree of movement during healing. These splints are generally left in place for 7 to 10 days. They use a variety of materials including orthodontic wires, nonrigid titanium splints, and enamel bonding material.

Options commonly available to emergency medicine providers for temporary splinting of reimplanted teeth include the use of periodontal pastes, self-cure composites, and composite adhered mesh ribbon (**Table 2**). A frequently used periodontal paste, COE-PAK, is available as 2 components, a base and a catalyst. When mixed together in ribbons of equal length, a pliable but sticky puttylike substance results. The clinician wears gloves kept moist with water to avoid sticking, and applies the COE-PAK to the involved tooth (or teeth) and onto the stable, uninjured teeth on either side, forming a splint that will hold the reimplanted teeth in place. To enhance adherence, the teeth and gingiva in the area to be covered should be dried with gauze or blown dry with air. The mixed COE-PAK is rolled into a cylinder and applied to the front (facial) surface of the involved teeth and gingiva including the area between the teeth. The material dries

Table 2	
Basic dental equipment for ED treatment of traumatic injury	
Material/Product	**Use**
Calcium hydroxide paste or Self-cure composite or light-cured composite	Coverage of fractures to dentin or pulp
Periodontal paste (COE-PAK) or Composite material and bondable ribbon	Splinting of loosened or replanted tooth
HBSS (eg, EMT Tooth Saver)	Storage of avulsed teeth
Bupivacaine with epinephrine	Dental anesthesia
Mixing pad and spatula	Preparation of compounds
Gauze rolls, tongue blades	Visualization and maintaining a dry field

and hardens, providing temporary support, but can be easily removed by a follow-up dental provider for more definitive splinting.

Other available splinting techniques recently discussed in the emergency medicine literature include the use of thin, meshlike, bondable ribbon or wire bonded to the teeth with composite resins that are cured (hardened) after exposure to a specialized light source. Although these techniques require specialized materials and equipment, as well as additional steps (etching the tooth surface with acid, application of an adhesive product and then a resin product), they have been shown to require skills that can be mastered by emergency physicians with limited training time. In an experimental model, although satisfaction with the end result was higher among dentist evaluators, the time required to perform the procedure was longer (8.8 vs 4.4 minutes on average) using these techniques.[16]

Additional treatments to be offered include the use of systemic antibiotics and pain medications, and updating tetanus immunization status as appropriate. Based on data extrapolated from animal studies, the use of oral antibiotics after reimplantation is recommended by recent dental association guidelines.[17,18] Human trials have been unable to show any significant effect of systemic antibiotics on the outcome of avulsed teeth reimplantation. A recent meta-analysis found the current literature to be inconclusive but the investigators recommended continued use pending further conclusive investigation.[19] Tetracycline is noted to be the antibiotic of choice because of its adjunctive effect on improving subsequent root resorption through an inherent negative effect on osteoclast function. it is administered as doxycycline (100 mg twice a day) for 7 days. In growing children at risk for tooth discoloration, or if otherwise contraindicated, penicillin VK (500 mg 4 times a day or 50 mg/kg/d divided 4 times a day) or clindamycin can be used.

After temporizing ED treatment, patients should be advised to follow up with a dental care provider as soon as possible for reevaluation and further care. Patients or parents should be informed that the prognosis for retention of the tooth is guarded and that further care and procedures by their dental follow-up provider will likely be inevitable.

SUBLUXATIONS AND LUXATIONS

Direct trauma to the dental structure may be of a force and angle resulting a loosening rather than dislodgement of the involved teeth.

Concussion refers to a tooth that has taken a blow and, although there may be some local pain and tenderness to percussion of the tooth, there is no increased mobility when the examiner palpates or attempts to manipulate the tooth crown. Although no specific therapy is required in this situation other than pain control if needed, the patient should be warned that there is a small chance of subsequent complications such as color change over the subsequent 10 to 14 days caused by pulp vessel injury[20] or tooth loss caused by subtle attachment apparatus injury.

The term subluxation refers to a tooth that is mobile in its socket but is not displaced from its normal position. Examination for location of the crown within the normal cascade of the patients' dentition as well as the patient's subjective sensation of a change in occlusion may be indications that a subtle change in position has occurred.

Luxation injury occurs when the involved tooth has experienced a change from its normal position within the socket. Luxation injuries are further divided into 4 types based on the position of the displaced tooth.

1. Intrusive luxation (intrusion): the tooth is displaced toward its apex or deeper onto the socket. The tooth appears shortened and may be so fully intruded that it

appears to be missing. Careful examination paired with radiographic studies may help to differentiate a fully intruded from an avulsed tooth.

2. Extrusive luxation: the tooth is forced out of the socket in a direction in line with the long axis of the tooth. The tooth appears elongated compared with its normal position.
3. Lateral luxation: the tooth is displaced either toward the labial side (facially), tongue side (lingually), more midline teeth (mesially), or more lateral teeth (distally).
4. Complete luxation (avulsion): the tooth is fully extruded from the socket as described earlier.

ED treatment considerations for subluxation and luxation injury depend primarily on the degree of mobility as well as the position of the injured tooth.

Teeth that are only minimally mobile on examination and maintained in a normal-appearing position do well with conservative management alone. No direct manipulation or stabilization attempt is indicated in the ED. The patient should be instructed to maintain a soft diet and avoid chewing directly on the involved tooth as much as possible for a period of 1 to 2 weeks. The patient should be instructed to seek dental follow-up at as early a date as possible and warned that there is some risk of discoloration or subsequent loss of the tooth because of injury to the attachment apparatus.

Teeth that are grossly mobile have a better chance of retention and survival if they are splinted in place temporarily pending dental follow-up. As previously described, there are several options for temporary dental splinting available to the emergency medicine practitioner. Periodontal paste such as COE-PAK is among the easiest and most widely available products to accomplish this goal. Remember that local anesthesia through the use of a periapical or other dental block technique may enhance patient comfort and cooperation during any splinting procedure.

Extruded or laterally luxated teeth should be realigned to as near a normal position as possible. Precise position need not be attained in the ED setting but relocating the tooth in the socket in as near to an anatomic position as possible both enhances patient comfort and allows an increased chance for the PDL and attachment apparatus to maintain physiologic conditions and survive. After providing local anesthesia with a periapical or other dental block to allow manipulation without undue discomfort, the position of the tooth should be adjusted to approximate its expected normal position. A temporary splinting material such as COE-PAK should then be applied.

Luxation injuries may involve fracture of the boney portion of the tooth socket or alveolar bone. Associated fractures in the tooth socket are difficult to detect in the ED setting but initial treatment is not affected by their presence. More widespread alveolar fractures should be suspected when there are several teeth in a section that are misaligned or loosened. Facial radiographs or panorex may show a fracture line just apical to the root of the teeth in the area; however, this may be difficult to see. Early repositioning and rigid splinting of the involved fracture fragment is the treatment of choice. Once identified by the emergency physician, consultation with oral surgeon or dentist, if available, is indicated to coordinate a treatment plan. Temporary alignment and splinting, as described earlier, may be indicated after such discussion while awaiting specialty evaluation.

Intruded teeth often are accompanied by an underlying alveolar bone or socket fracture as well as a crush-type injury and disruption of the attachment apparatus. These factors create a higher incidence of pulp necrosis and root resorption than is seen in other luxation injuries. These teeth are typically immobile in their intruded location and require neither repositioning nor splinting in the ED setting. Pain control and referral to dental care within 24 hours if possible are the recommended ED care. Permanent teeth are generally repositioning and likely will need root canal or other endodontic treatment. Primary teeth are often observed for a period to allow spontaneous reeruption.[5]

TOOTH FRACTURES

Trauma to the teeth may result not only in loosening or displacement of the tooth but also to breakage of the tooth structure. Fractures may involve only the visible portion of the tooth (crown) or extend into the tooth root. Initial treatment of these injuries depends primarily on the depth of the fracture line.

Various systems of nomenclature of crown fractures based on depth of involvement exist, with the Ellis classification often being used in emergency medicine texts (**Table 3**). However, this particular naming convention is not widely used by dental clinicians. Dental literature commonly classifies crown fractures as complicated if pulp is exposed and as uncomplicated if it is not. Initial care strategy differs within the uncomplicated class of fractures based on involvement of dentin. To avoid confusion, thinking of and describing crown fractures based on a physical description of the depth of involvement is recommended.

Examination of teeth that have undergone fracture should include careful visual inspection after cleaning off any associated blood or foreign material. Examination of the fracture area as described later to determine the depth of injury should be accompanied by gentle rocking of the tooth to assess for any subluxation injury. Exposure of the tooth to cool water or gentle blowing of forced air, such as is available from a compressed air or oxygen source, can help to assess for sensitivity.

Cracking of the enamel surface with no loss of material (infraction) is generally not associated with any pain or sensitivity of the involved tooth. No emergent intervention is required; however, the patient should be referred to a dentist for follow-up. Dentists sometimes apply a covering to the tooth surface to prevent subsequent staining of the enamel. In addition, the patient should be reminded that there is a small chance of subsequent tooth discoloration or other complications as described earlier.

Fractures that involve only the enamel of the tooth are characterized by loss of some portion of the normal contour of the tooth edge. The base of the fracture area has an appearance consistent with the color and sheen of the typical tooth enamel. There is no exposure of the more yellow tinged or porous appearance characteristic of dentin. These injuries typically do not cause sensitivity to temperature or forced air. Rough edges of the fracture may be uncomfortable for the patient and represent a potential for injury to the tongue or lip mucosa. Smoothing of these sharp edges may be carried out with an emery board but otherwise no specific immediate treatment is necessary. The patient should be referred for timely dental follow-up. Restoration of the normal contours of the tooth can be accomplished using composite resins for aesthetic purposes. Although this degree of injury represents a minimal risk to the viability of

Table 3
Classification of dental crown fractures

Descriptive Classification	Ellis Classification	Dental Literature Classification
Enamel cracks (no loss of enamel)	—	Infraction
Fracture enamel only (no dentin exposed)	Ellis class I	Uncomplicated crown fracture
Fracture involving dentin (no pulp exposed)	Ellis class II	
Fracture involving pulp	Ellis class III	Complicated crown fracture

the tooth, rare (<1%) occurrence of subsequent color change and pulp necrosis has been cited in the dental literature.

Fractures that extend into the dentin of the tooth are at higher risk for subsequent inflammation or infection of the pulp cavity leading to necrosis and tooth loss. Dentin contains a microtubular structure that makes it porous, allowing access for intraoral microbial flora to the deeper structures of the tooth. These fractures are recognized by appearance: 2 different layers of material with more yellow dentin at the base of the fracture. The tooth is sensitive to temperature and forced air exposure. Initial treatment goals are to provide an appropriate covering of the exposed dentin to limit risk of ongoing contamination and to provide pain relief. Risk of subsequent complications increases related to both the depth of the fracture (more proximity to the pulp) and the time from injury to fracture coverage, thus making timely care in the ED important if immediate dental follow-up is not available.

Suitable material for coverage of fractures provides an adequate barrier to contamination without causing inflammation. Various materials have been used for this purpose, including calcium hydroxide (CaOH), zinc oxide, and glass ionomer composites.

To allow preparation of the tooth and dressing application, it is recommended that supraperiosteal periapical block or regional dental anesthesia be performed before the procedure.

One of the most commonly available options found in the ED is CaOH paste. CaOH is available premixed or as 2 components, a base and a catalyst. Equal amounts of the 2 should be mixed on a nonporous surface such as a mixing pad using a dental spatula or other instrument. The mixture should then be applied to the dried surface of the involved tooth fracture. It adheres and hardens over a few minutes. Although coverage of the CaOH bandage with foil to provide a further occlusal barrier is classically described, this can be difficult to keep in place and is thought not to be necessary if further follow-up is possible within the next 24 to 36 hours.[21]

Pain control should be prescribed. The patient should be instructed to eat only soft foods and avoid any chewing on the fracture area. Prompt follow-up with the dentist should be recommended.

These fractures have an increased rate of subsequent pulp necrosis and other complications (10%) and patients should be warned that, despite appropriate ED treatment, root canal or other endodontic treatment is often required. Dentists can frequently restore a normal appearance to the tooth with composite materials and may either remove or incorporate the initial dressing material placed for initial coverage.

Fractures that extend into the pulp of the tooth are characterized by visualization of the pink pulp material at the base of the defect. Although typically painful and sensitive to temperature and forced air, concussion of the nerve from the initial injury may result in a tooth that is insensate at the time of initial examination. Direct exposure of the pulp to infection and inflammatory substances creates a high risk of resulting pulp necrosis in these injuries. Immediate referral to dental care providers is indicated, if possible, for consideration of endodontic procedures. If emergent evaluation by a dental provider is not feasible, coverage of the fracture site as described earlier is recommended, because this prevents further bacterial contamination and mitigates pain once the dental block wears off. Pain control and evaluation by a dentist as soon as possible is recommended, with protection of the area from chewing in the interim.

Systemic antibiotic use in tooth fractures, although cited in some sources, is not currently recommended. Although dentin or pulp exposure creates a potential portal of entry for oral flora, there have been no studies showing a significant negative effect on outcomes caused by infection. There have been no human studies suggesting a benefit of antibiotic administration on crown or crown-root fracture in humans.[22]

MANDIBLE FRACTURES

The mandible, the only mobile bone of the maxillofacial structure, is a U-shaped bone articulating with the skull at the TMJs. Fractures are typically described by location within one of 6 anatomic regions within the mandible structure. The symphysis or parasymphyseal area describes that portion of the mandible spanning from one mandibular canine tooth to the other. The body of the mandible, that area from the posterior aspect of the canine tooth to the posterior aspect of the second molar, is the most common area of fracture in adults.[23] The angle starts posterior to the second molar and becomes the area of the ramus, where it takes on a more vertical orientation. The coronoid process is the protuberance anterior to the sigmoid notch and is rarely fractured in isolation. The condyle is composed of the neck region and the head, which forms the articulation with the temporal bone. As with any other fracture a description of the location, degree of comminution and the direction and amount of any displacement, as well as whether the fracture is open or closed, will aid in planning when discussed with the consultant. Open fractures generally manifest with intraoral gingival lacerations and bleeding.

The typical mechanism of injury causing fractures of the mandible involve either a forced occlusion, such as a fall striking the chin, often resulting in injury to the TMJ or the condyle area, or a blow from the lateral or frontolateral direction resulting in body or angle fractures.

As with other facial bone fractures, the incidence of mandibular fracture in young children is lower than that in adolescents and adults. This is thought to be related to a combination of factors including elasticity of the bony structures, stabilization of the mandible by unerupted secondary teeth, and a large cranial versus facial anatomy resulting in the force of blows often primarily impacting the skull and forehead areas.[24] However, when they do occur, mandible fractures in the pediatric population raise special considerations both during initial care and in follow-up. The younger age group (0–4 years of age) seems to have an increased incidence of significant associated injuries likely because of the higher degree of force necessary to cause the fracture.[24,25] These injuries include both skull fracture and brain injury and significant facial soft tissue injury. Associated cervical spine injury, although still infrequent, occurred in 3.3% of hospitalized pediatric patients with trauma with facial fractures versus only 1.3% of those without facial bony injury.[24] Although no specific recommendations regarding evaluation can be made from these data, consideration must be given to careful screening for associated injuries in this age group. Although primarily a concern for follow-up providers, parents should be warned that fractures in the 4-year-old to 11-year-old age group have been associated in up to 22% of cases with later facial bone growth abnormalities requiring secondary surgical procedures.[26] Fracture lines that involve the buds of developing permanent teeth may result in difficulty with development of adult dentition.[27]

Classic teaching holds that the arched shape of the mandible transmits forces in such a way that fractures frequently occur in more than one area of the U. Fractures may occur remote from and on the side opposite the point of impact. Typical bilateral injury patterns include bilateral condyle fractures, bilateral angle fractures, bilateral body fractures, and fracture of the mandible body combined with a contralateral angle fracture (**Table 4**). Although multiple fractures may be present and should be carefully sought, a study based on computed tomography (CT) imaging has shown that up to

Table 4			
Incidence of mandible fractures by location			
Common Fractures (%)		Uncommon Fractures (%)	
Condyle	36	Ramus	3
Body	21	Coronoid process	3
Angle	20	Alveolar ridge	3
Symphysis	14	—	—

42% of mandible fractures may be unifocal.[28] One theory holds that unifocal fractures may result when some of the force of impact is dissipated by injury, such as subluxation, at the TMJ. However, only a minority (16%) of those with unifocal fracture had evidence of such injury in this study.

Because of the traction of attached muscles, mandibular fractures are often displaced. Symphyseal fractures that run obliquely through the mandible and bilateral body fractures are frequently pulled posteriorly. Fractures through the angle may result in the posterior portion of the mandible being pulled superiorly.[29]

EVALUATION

As discussed earlier, mandibular fractures and associated oral or facial injuries have an impact on airway patency and support. After evaluating and necessary treatment of more severe injury, initial examination should include visual inspection for areas of swelling or asymmetry of the jaw as well as observation for a normal range of motion. Limitation in mouth opening with a maximum distance of less than 5 cm between the incisors may indicate fracture.[28] Premature contact of the molars with an inability to fully close the front teeth may indicate a subcondylar fracture on that side. Lateral deviation of the jaw either at rest or with attempted opening should also be sought. Palpate the mandible for areas of tenderness or step-off, including in the region of the TMJ. Assess and document the area of the chin and lower lip in the distribution of the mental nerve to light touch sensation. Fractures through the anterior portion of the body of the mandible can affect this branch of the inferior alveolar nerve through its course within the mandible or as it exits at the mental foramen.

Intraoral examination for hematoma and gingival bleeding or laceration should be carried out. Palpation of the mandibular dentition may reveal loosening or step-off of a block of teeth, indicating an alveolar ridge fracture or a through-and-through mandibular fracture.

In the awake, cooperative patient, a subjective sense of a change in occlusion can provide an important clue to possible fracture and is more sensitive than clinicians' impressions of such an abnormality.[28] Subjective malocclusion had a sensitivity of 75% and specificity of 96% and seemed to be the best single indicator in one of the few studies designed to prospectively assess findings that suggested mandible fracture.[30]

Among patients with trauma to the area of the mandible, various studies have shown that only 25% to 40% have fracture.[31,32] No single clinical finding has been found to accurately rule out fracture. A study of patients with suspected mandibular fracture from the United Kingdom suggests that a clinical decision rule based on the absence of malocclusion, trismus, dental fracture, a palpable or visible step-off, or subjective pain with the mouth closed was able to predict patients in whom no fracture was present on radiograph (**Box 1**). Sensitivity was 100%, specificity was 39%, and application of the rule could reduce radiograph use by 31%.[31]

Box 1
Decision rule for imaging suspected mandible fractures
The Manchester Mandibular Fracture Decision Rule
1. Do the patient's teeth meet abnormally?
2. Can the patient open the mouth normally?
3. Are there any broken teeth present?
4. Any report of pain with the mouth closed?
5. Is there a step off deformity?
If yes to any of the above mandibular xrays obtained.
From Busuito MJ, Smith DJ, Robson MC. Mandibular fractures in an urban trauma center. J Trauma 1986;26:826–9; with permission.

The tongue blade test (TBT) is another tool that can be used in screening to determine the likelihood of mandibular fracture and need for further radiographic evaluation. Useful in patients who are awake and cooperative and in whom other intraoral injury such as soft tissue laceration or tooth trauma does not cause pain limiting the patient's bite, 2 variations have been described.

In the first technique, a wooden tongue depressor is held between the teeth and the patient is asked to hold it in place while the examiner tries to pull it out. The test is performed on both sides of the mouth with the inability to keep it in place on either side deemed a positive test. In a study of 110 patients, using what was described as an otherwise undefined mild traction force, the TBT had a sensitivity of 95%, a specificity of 67%, and a negative predictive value of 96%.[30]

A second technique involves the tongue blade being held in the teeth while the examiner applies a twisting motion. The ability of the patient to maintain the bite until enough force is applied to crack the tongue blade is the expected norm. Using this method, similar results have been obtained, with a sensitivity of 96%, a specificity of 64%, and a negative predictive value for fracture of 95%.[33]

RADIOGRAPHIC EVALUATION

Options for radiographic evaluation of the mandible include plain film radiographs, panoramic tomography (panorex), and CT scan. Plain film series consists of multiple views in an attempt to isolate areas of the mandible.[20] Typical views and the areas they best evaluate include posteroanterior view (rami and body) (**Fig. 1**), Towne view (condyles, rami, and TMJ), (**Fig. 2**) and bilateral oblique views (body and angle) (**Fig. 3**). These multiple views require significant positioning that may not be feasible in patients who are otherwise injured or may be unable to cooperate. Designed to eliminate the overlap of soft tissues and bony structures from the radiograph, panorex films are obtained using specific equipment that allows rotation of the x-ray tube and film cassette about the patients head. Although generally considered more sensitive for visualizing fractures, especially in the area of the rami and condyles, published evidence suggests only a modest advantage compared with plain films.[34,35] Many EDs may not have this specific equipment available. In addition, the patient must be able to sit upright for such views to be obtained. Given the difficulty in obtaining these films and in interpreting bony facial anatomy because of multiple overlapping shadows, CT has become the imaging study of choice for most cases of maxillofacial

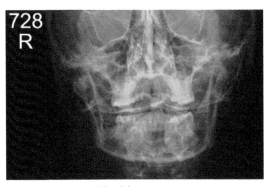

Fig. 1. Posteroanterior view (rami and body).

trauma.[55] However, in the case of isolated mandibular trauma, some surgeons have continued to prefer plain films and panorex images.[36] Although several older studies using a resolution based on 3-mm slices suggested that CT may have a lower sensitivity than panorex imaging, newer scan protocols using higher resolution 1-mm slices were seen to outperform other modalities and have 100% sensitivity.[37] Images obtained by CT scan often provide better visualization of the fracture (**Fig. 4**), and the ability to perform reconstructions allows more exact characterization of these often multisite fractures (**Fig. 5**).

One suggested approach is to use plain films for initial screening if the patient is able to cooperate with the required positioning. CT scan can be performed if suspicion is high but initial films fail to reveal fracture. If available and appropriate to patient condition, panorex should be substituted for plain film series as the initial study. In cases in which positioning is difficult or CT scans are already being performed for other indications, forgoing initial plain films is suggested.

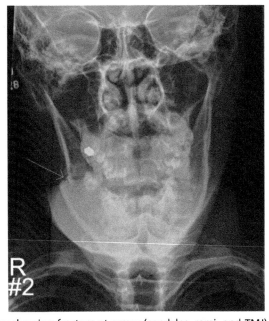

Fig. 2. Towne view showing fracture at arrow (condyles, rami, and TMJ).

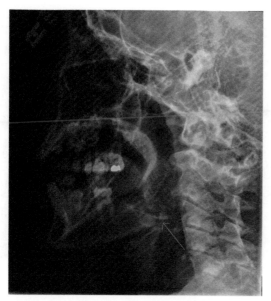

Fig. 3. Oblique view of the mandible showing fracture at arrow (body and angle).

TREATMENT

Treatment options depend on the location and degree of displacement of the fracture as well as the age of the patient and status of dentition. Options range from observation and maintaining a soft diet to open reduction with internal fixation. The placement of arch bars secured to the teeth with maxillomandibular fixation (MMF) is the most frequent splinting technique used.[38] In patients with poor underlying dental structures or in the edentulous patient, this may not be feasible. Along with significant

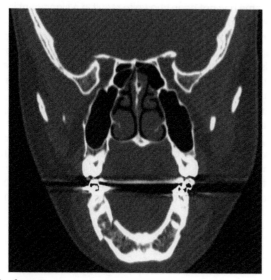

Fig. 4. CT scan of a fracture.

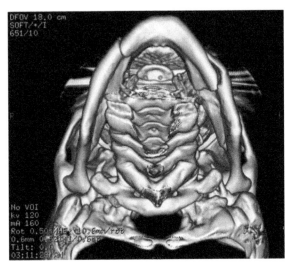

Fig. 5. Reconstruction of multisite fractures.

displacement or instability of fracture fragments, these issues are indications for operative fixation, which is generally accomplished via an intraoral or submental approach.[36]

After identification of fractures, specialty consultation with oromaxillofacial surgeons; ear, nose, and throat; or other appropriate services should be obtained to discuss the details and timing of the next treatment step. Open fractures require antibiotic therapy providing coverage of intraoral flora, typically penicillin, cephalosporins,[39] or clindamycin. Pain control and tetanus status should be addressed as needed.

Definitive treatment of mandible fractures need not be performed on an emergent basis. Although intervention within 24 to 48 hours is typically recommended, delay beyond this time frame has not been shown to result in a significant increase in complications.[40,41] In the absence of other injuries requiring admission, patients with nondisplaced, closed fractures may be discharged for timely follow-up that has been specifically arranged with a specialist. Elective operative repair or further fixation can be accomplished as an outpatient procedure. Liquids-only versus a soft diet and nil-by-mouth status for planned next day intervention are best discussed on a case-by-case basis with the follow-up provider.

Mandible fractures in the pediatric population represent several specific considerations both at the time of injury and in ongoing follow-up. Initial treatment options may be altered because primary dentition may not provide enough stability to support maxillomandibular fixation. Longer term complications may result from associated injury to the secondary dentition germinal buds or from deleterious effect on future bone growth resulting either from the initial fracture or from operative intervention.[42] Consultation with and referral to a provider comfortable with these factors is critical.

SUMMARY

Traumatic injury to the teeth, their supporting structures, and the mandible are frequently encountered in the practice of emergency medicine. Proper diagnosis and prompt, appropriate temporizing treatment plays a crucial role in optimizing the long-term outcome for patients with these injuries. Emergency physicians should be comfortable with the initial evaluation and management strategies discussed in this article.

REFERENCES

1. Hieawy A, Taher D. Luxation dental injuries: review of treatment guidelines and endodontic considerations. J Emergency Medicine Trauma and Acute Care 2006;6(2):3–7.
2. Benko K. Dental pain. In: Mahadevan SV, Garmel GM, editors. An introduction to clinical emergency medicine. 2nd edition. Cambridge (MA): Cambridge University Press; 2012. p. 255–8.
3. A costly dental destination. The Pew center on the states Web site. Available at: http://pewtrusts.org. Accessed December 16, 2012.
4. Guidelines on the management of acute dental trauma. 2011 revision. American Academy of Pediatric Dentistry Web site. Available at: http://www.aapd.org/. Accessed July 19, 2011.
5. Nazif M, Martin BS, McKibben DH, et al. Oral disorders. In: Zitelli BJ, Davis HW, editors. Atlas of pediatric physical diagnosis. 5th edition. Philadelphia: Mosby; 2007. p. 755–70, 776–7.
6. Wright JT. Anatomy and development of the teeth; Up to date Web site. version 19.2. Available at: http://www.uptodate.com. Accessed September 25, 2011.
7. American Dental Association Web site. Available at: http://www.ada.org. Accessed September 21, 2011.
8. Walls RM, Vissers RJ. The traumatized airway. In: Hagberg CA, editor. Benumof's airway management: principles and practice. 2nd edition. Philadelphia: Mosby Elsevier; 2001. p. 946–7.
9. Andreasen JO, Andreasen FM. Avulsions. In: Andreasen JO, Andreasen FM, Andersson L, editors. Textbook and color atlas of traumatic injuries to the teeth. 4th edition. Oxford (United Kingdom): Wiley-Blackwell; 2007. p. 444.
10. Lin S, Zuckerman O, Fuss Z, et al. New emphasis in the treatment of dental trauma: avulsions and luxations. Dent Traumatol 2007. http://dx.doi.org/10.1111/j.1600-9657.2005.00455x.
11. Souza B, Luckemeyer D, et al. Effect of temperature and storage media on human periodontal ligament fibroblast viability. Dent Traumatol 2010;26:271–5.
12. Trope M. Clinical management of the avulsed tooth: present strategies and future directions. Dent Traumatol 2002;18:1–11.
13. Amsterdam JT, Kilgore KP. Regional anesthesia of the head and neck. In: Roberts JR, Hedges JR, editors. Clinical procedures in emergency medicine. 5th edition. Philadelphia: Saunders; 2010. p. 500–9.
14. McIntyre J, et al. Management of avulsed permanent incisors: a comprehensive update. Pediatr Dent 2007;29(1):56–63.
15. Ma KM, Sae-Lim V. The effect of topical minocycline on replacement resorption of replanted monkeys' teeth. Dent Traumatol 2003;19:96–102.
16. McIntosh MS, Konzelmann J, Smith J, et al. Stabilization and treatment of dental avulsions and fractures by emergency physicians using just-in-time training. Ann Emerg Med 2009;54(4):585–92.
17. Recommended guidelines of the American Association of Endodontists for traumatic dental injuries. American Association of Endodontists Web site. Revised Oct 2004. Available at: http://aae.org/. Accessed August 14, 2012.

18. Dental trauma guidelines. International Association of Dental Traumatology Web site. Revised 2011. Available at: http://www.iadt-dentaltrauma.org/. Accessed December 16, 2012.
19. Hinckfuss SE, Messer LB. An evidence-based assessment of the clinical guidelines for replanted avulsed teeth. Part II: prescription of systemic antibiotics. Dent Traumatol 2009;25(2):158–64.
20. Flores C, Schwartz DT. Facial radiology. In: Schwartz DT, Reisdorff EJ, editors. Emergency radiology. New York: McGraw-Hill; 2000. p. 349–61.
21. Benko K. Emergency dental procedures. In: Roberts JR, Hedges JR, editors. Clinical procedures in emergency medicine. 5th edition. Philadelphia: Saunders; 2010. p. 1220–2.
22. Andreasen JO, Jensen SS, Sae-Lim V. The role of antibiotics in preventing healing complications after traumatic dental injuries: a literature review. Endodontic Topics 2006;14:80–92.
23. Avery L, Susaria S, Noveline R. Multidetector and three-dimensional CT evaluation of the patient with maxillofacial injury. Radiol Clin North Am 2011;49(1): 183–203.
24. Imahara SD, Hopper RA, Wang J, et al. Patterns and outcomes of pediatric facial fractures in the United States: a survey of the national trauma data bank. J Am Coll Surg 2008;207(5):710–6.
25. Infante CP, Espin Galvez F, et al. A retrospective study of 99 fractures in 59 patients. Int J Oral Maxillofac Surg 1994;23:329.
26. Demianczuk AN, Verchere C, Phillips JH. The effect on facial growth of pediatric mandibular fractures. J Craniofac Surg 1999;10(4):323–8.
27. Ratan R, Ylipaavalneiemi P. The effect of jaw fractures in children on the development of permanent teeth and the occlusion. Proc Finn Dent Soc 1973;69:99–104.
28. Escott EJ, Bransetter BF. Incidence and characterization of unifocal mandible fractures on CT. AJNR Am J Neuroradiol 2008;29:890–4.
29. Cail WS. Face. In: Keats TE, editor. Emergency radiology. 2nd edition. Chicago: Year Book Medical; 1989. p. 47–55.
30. Schwab RA, Genners K, Robinson WA. Clinical predictors of mandible fractures. Am J Emerg Med 1998;16(3):304–5.
31. Busuito MJ, Smith DJ, Robson MC. Mandibular fractures in an urban trauma centre. J Trauma 1986;26:826–9.
32. Charalambous C, Dunnig J, Omorphos S, et al. A maximally sensitive clinical decision rule to reduce the need for radiography in mandibular trauma. Ann R Coll Surg Engl 2005;87:259–63.
33. Alonso LA, Purcell TB. Accuracy of the tongue blade test in patients with suspected mandibular fracture. J Emerg Med 1995;13:297–304.
34. Guss DA, Clark RF, Peitz T, et al. Pantomography vs mandibular series for the detection of mandibular fractures. Acad Emerg Med 2000;7(2):141–5.
35. Mackway-Jones K. Towards evidence based emergency medicine: Best BETs from the Manchester Royal Infirmary. J Accid Emerg Med 2000;17:46–9.
36. Kellman RM. Maxillofacial trauma. In: Flint PW, Haughey BH, Lund VJ, et al, editors. Cummings otolaryngology: head & neck surgery. 5th edition. Philadelphia: Mosby; 2010. p. 318–40.
37. Wilson IF, Lokeh A, Benjamin CU, et al. Prospective comparison of panoramic tomography (zonography) and helical computed tomography in the diagnosis and management of mandibular fractures. Plast Reconstr Surg 2001;107(6):1369–75.
38. McKay MP, Mayersak RJ. Facial trauma. In: Marx JA, editor. Rosen's emergency medicine. 7th edition. Philadelphia: Mosby; 1999. p. 335–7.

39. Heit JM, Stevens MR, Jeffords K. Comparison of ceftriaxone with penicillin for antibiotic prophylaxis for compound mandible fractures. Oral Surg Oral Med Oral Pathol Oral Radiol Endod 1997;83(4):423–6.
40. Lucca M, Shastri K, McKenzie W, et al. Comparison of treatment outcomes associated with early vs late treatment of mandible fractures: a retrospective chart review and analysis. J Oral Maxillofac Surg 2010;68(10):2484–8.
41. Barker DA, Park SS. Is fixation of mandible fractures urgent? Laryngoscope 2011; 121:906–7.
42. Krakovitz PR, Koltal PJ. Pediatric facial fractures. In: Flint PW, Haughey BH, Lund VJ, et al, editors. Cummings otolaryngology: head & neck surgery. 5th edition. Philadelphia: Mosby; 2010. p. 2699–715.

Index

Note: Page numbers of article titles are in **boldface** type.

Emerg Med Clin N Am 31 (2013) 575–581
http://dx.doi.org/10.1016/S0733-8627(13)00025-4
0733-8627/13/$ – see front matter © 2013 Elsevier Inc. All rights reserved.

emed.theclinics.com

mergencyMed **Advancé**

ll the latest emergency medicine news and research you need, all in one place

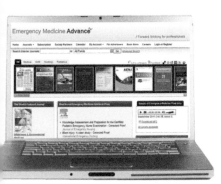

EmergencyMedAdvance.com is a new essential online resource offering valued high-quality content and news for the global community of Emergency Medicine professionals to save time and stay current—from physicians and nurses to EMTs.

ay current
Emergency Medicine news

ve time
Access relevant articles in press from 16 participating journals

nd more...
ournals' profiles
Personalized search results
Emergency Medicine bookstore

- Upcoming meetings and events

- Search across 500+ health sciences journals
- Learn how to submit a manuscript

- Sign up for free e-Alerts
- Emergency Medicine jobs

**ookmark us today at
mergencyMedAdvance.com**

Printed and bound by CPI Group (UK) Ltd, Croydon, CR0 4YY

03/10/2024

01040439-0020